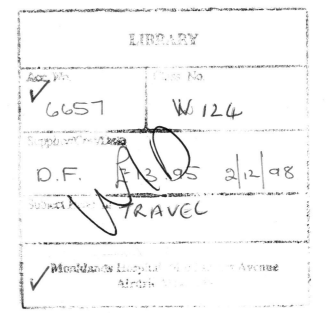

ABC OF HEALTHY TRAVEL

Fifth edition

ABC OF HEALTHY TRAVEL

Fifth edition

ERIC WALKER FRCP MRCGP

Consultant Physician/Epidemiologist
Scottish Centre for Infection and Environmental Health, Ruchill Hospital, Glasgow

GLYN WILLIAMS MRCP DTM&H

Consultant Physician
Cross House Hospital, Kilmarnock

FIONA RAESIDE BA RGN RM

Research Sister
Scottish Centre for Infection and Environmental Health, Ruchill Hospital, Glasgow

LORNA CALVERT RGN MN

Travel Health and Immunisation Nurse Specialist
Scottish Centre for Infection and Environmental Health, Ruchill Hospital, Glasgow

BMJ
Publishing
Group

British Library Cataloguing in Publication Data
A catalogue record for this book is available from the British Library

First edition 1983
Second edition 1985
Third edition November 1989
Second impression 1992
Fourth edition 1993
Fifth edition 1997

ISBN: 0-7279-1138-4

Typeset in Great Britain by Apek Typesetters Ltd, Nailsea, Avon
Printed in Great Britain at Cambridge University Press, Cambridge

Contents

Acknowledgements

We are grateful to the following for their help in the preparation of this book: Dr S Bhattacharji, Dr R J Crawford, Dr H Datta, Dr J P Delamere, Mr R Dewar, Dr E A C Follett, Professor H M Gilles, Professor N R Grist, Dr S Ighedosa, Dr E H McLaren, Mrs D Moran, Dr D Reid, Dr R T A Scott, Dr J C M Sharp, Miss Edith H Simpson, Mr D Sutherland, Mrs Sheila J Thomson, Dr P J Watkins, Mrs E Wilson, Dr R Wilcox.

TRAVEL MEDICINE AND PROBLEMS FACING THE TRAVELLER

Why travel medicine?

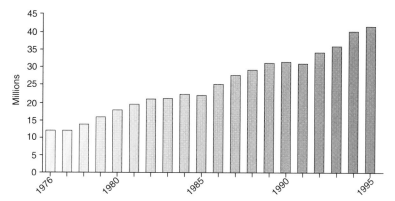

Travellers leaving Britain for visits overseas each year.

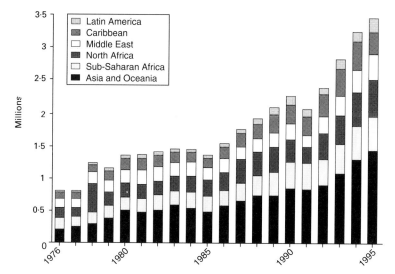

Travellers leaving Britain to visit areas with increased risk of infection.

The specialty of travel medicine has developed in response to the enormous increase in international travel over the past 20–30 years. This increase and the speed of travel has brought into question the traditional geographical concept of "tropical" disease. We talk now of "emerging and re-emerging" diseases with, for example, malaria presenting worldwide and "diseases of development" such as diabetes mellitus being common in Africa and Asia. Worldwide concern develops overnight when there is an outbreak of haemorrhagic fever or plague that has the potential to be rapidly carried between continents. HIV infection has taken only 20 years to spread throughout the world, which would have been inconceivable 100 years ago.

In addition there are problems specific to rapid travel, such as jetlag, accidents, unaccustomed exposure to sun, cold, altitude, and encounters with very different cultures. Extreme economic differences between host countries and visitors can lead to accidents from driving in poorly maintained vehicles on rough roads, to tourists being isolated within compounds because of the danger of mugging, and the growth of "sex tourism" with its attendant health risks.

These changes have led health care specialists throughout the world to focus on the special needs of travellers and increasingly also on the associated needs of the host countries.

Travel medicine is an interdisciplinary specialty combining prevention skills, public health, research, education, and clinical care. Courses, qualifications, and societies are described in the final chapter.

Travel medicine also responds to the need for continual surveillance and research which enables sensible decisions to be made, for example, on the need for specific vaccinations. The growth in electronic communications allows rapid exchange of information about disease risks, outbreaks of infection, and local public health requirements. One of the challenges is to collect together this information and to provide useful and continually updated health information to travellers, usually through their general practitioner and, increasingly, the practice nurse. On-line databases, regularly updated wall charts, and postgraduate education courses are all ways of achieving this.

What is the problem?

The numbers of people travelling on "package tours" to Mediterranean countries continue to increase, and holidays in tropical areas such as East Africa and Asia are now commonplace. In 1995, 40m visits were taken abroad by people living in Britain. Businesses, missionary societies, and "service overseas" schemes may have several hundreds of people overseas at any time, some on short trips, others staying for many years. Air travel has enabled people to visit relatives both for holidays and at short notice to help with family crises. All these groups go through the upheaval of leaving familiar surroundings and having to cope with unexpected circumstances. Their health may not be protected by services and legislation well established at home. Changes in food and water may bring unexpected problems, as may insects and insect borne diseases, especially in hot countries. Few have at their fingertips the current detailed knowledge needed to advise the traveller going to a particular country, and personal reminiscences may not always reflect current or common problems. A danger of generalising is that it may be forgotten, for example, that malaria is a risk in parts of Turkey, diphtheria has recently increased in Russia, and hepatitis A virus, of worldwide distribution, is not destroyed by many methods of purifying drinking water.

In transit

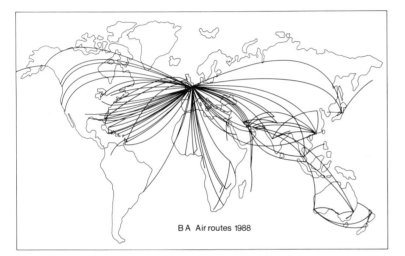

B A Air routes 1988

An unpredictable environment is a problem for the overland traveller who plans his or her own journey, and greater knowledge of disease prevention and its management is needed than by the traveller in an aeroplane or on a sea cruise, whose environment, food, and drink are largely in the hands of the operator. Unforeseen changes in timetables may lead to stays in accommodation not of the expected standard. Delays at airports where the facilities have not kept pace with increased demand can be in overcrowded and unhygienic conditions, and also insect borne diseases may be contracted. Jetlag and exhaustion may prompt a traveller to take risks with food and drink.

While abroad

The most common illnesses occuring in travellers overseas

Sunburn
Diarrhoea and vomiting
Minor physical injuries
Skin infections
Alcohol related disease

The most common reasons for emergency repatriation on medical grounds

Ischaemic heart disease
Cerebrovascular accidents
Road traffic and other physical injuries
Psychiatric illness

More experienced travellers tend to have fewer health problems. Better planning, immunisations, and experience in prevention may all play a part, as well as salutary lessons learnt on previous occasions.

Surveys of returning travellers show that many have diarrhoea or respiratory symptoms while abroad. Excessive alcohol, sun, and late nights add to their problems. About 1 in 100 package holidaymakers who take out a health insurance policy make a claim. Diarrhoea and sunburn are principal reasons but accidents are also common. Injuries occur in and around swimming pools, to pedestrians forgetting that traffic drives on the right, and from unfamiliar equipment such as gates on lifts. Sexually transmitted diseases and AIDS are real risks throughout the world for those who take part in high risk activities. Those with pre-existing health problems may need to take special care and seek advice before travelling.

Long stay travellers may adapt to initial problems but then find themselves contracting diseases endemic in their chosen country, such as malaria, hepatitis, diarrhoea, and skin problems. Poliomyelitis would be common if most travellers were not effectively immunised. In some countries road traffic accidents are a major cause of morbidity and mortality, with unmetalled roads, poorly maintained vehicles, including motor bikes, alcohol, and unpredictable driving all playing a part. Some emotional problems, and problems of culture shock, may be resolved only by an early return home.

Insurance and medical services overseas

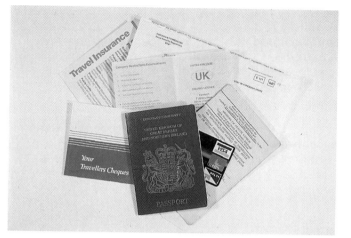

Some important travel documents. A copy of passport details speeds up replacement if it is lost.

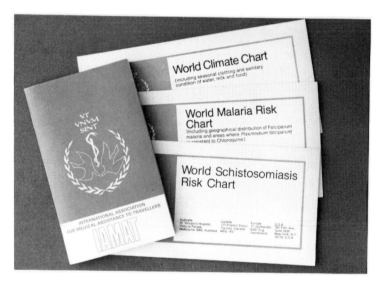

The traveller should be insured against medical expenses, and most policies include the cost of flying the sick person home when appropriate. Such insurance, however, rarely covers a service overseas similar to that available at home. Language and administrative differences are likely. Leaflet T5, issued by the Department of Health, describes the free or reduced cost medical treatments available in countries outside the European Community with reciprocal health arrangements, and the documents (passport, NHS medical card, certificate) which the traveller may have to carry. Leaflet T5 also gives details about arrangements within the European Community and an application form for certificate E111, which some countries require. Reciprocal arrangements between countries differ and money may have to be paid and then reclaimed in the visited country itself, which can be time consuming. Consultations with doctors may be free but not medication. Extra provision should be made for such emergencies.

Only a "small" supply of drugs for personal use may be taken out of Britain unless Home Office permission is obtained.

It can be important to find out about local medical services and the availability of essential drugs before setting out. This is especially important for those with disabilities or illnesses prone to unexpected crises, such as diabetes mellitus, those with children going to remote areas, the elderly or those pregnant. Friends, tour companies, British embassies and consulates overseas, and associations such as the International Association for Medical Assistance to Travellers are possible sources of advice.

It is wise for travellers to have a dental check up before departure to avoid unnecessary suffering and expense (insurance policies may not cover dental care) and to take spare spectacles and a current lens prescription.

After returning

Some important infections which can be contracted by travellers

Traveller's diarrhoea due to *E. coli*, Shigella, Salmonella and Campylobacter
Respiratory tract infections, "colds", influenza, Legionnaires' disease

Giardiasis	Malaria
Amoebiasis	Hepatitis A and E
Enteric fever	Hepatitis B
Schistosomiasis	HIV infection
Intestinal helminths	Onchocerciasis
Tick borne typhus	Tuberculosis
Dengue	Diphtheria

With the speed of air travel almost all communicable diseases may be in the incubation phase when the traveller returns home. Important examples are malaria, typhoid, cholera, and viral haemorrhagic fever. The actual numbers of imported diseases, measured by notification and laboratory returns, have increased. Malaria and intestinal infections are typical examples. General practitioners and casualty officers need to be aware of this and may need to seek specialist advice early in an illness, even years after the travellers' return. "When were you last abroad?" is an important question to ask when taking a history, particularly if fever, diarrhoea, jaundice, or skin rashes are present.

A check list for the surgery

- Are routine immunisations recommended at home up to date?
- What are the legal requirements for the countries being visited and what other immunisations are currently recommended by those with special knowledge of the risks?
- Are there special visa requirements, such as proof of a negative HIV test, as a condition of entry—usually only for long stay travellers.
- Is malarial infection possible? The Department of Health issues information in Leaflet T5 available free of charge from post offices. The most appropriate prophylactic drug can vary from year to year and advice can be sought from one of the centres listed in the chapter on malaria.
- What other advice is necessary so that the travellers can avoid infections such as HIV, schistosomiasis, and insect borne diseases such as dengue, typhus, and filariasis?
- Does your patient have any special health requirements?

Sources of up-to-date advice include

- T5 leaflet for the public from UK post offices
- Department of Health—"green book" on immunisation and "yellow book" on overseas travel for health care professionals
- Charts for the surgery, e.g. in *Practice Nurse, Doctor* and *Pulse*
- Online databases—TRAVAX and MASTA
- Telephone advice for health care professionals from specialist centres

---

SPECIAL CATEGORIES OF TRAVELLERS

The business traveller

Business travel is becoming increasingly common and poses its own challenges and problems. Some large companies which send many travellers abroad are now beginning to realise the benefits of travel preparation for their employees and have well-organised occupational health departments with suitably trained doctors and nurses. Unfortunately, most companies do not have this sort of provision, and often the business traveller is sent along to the GP or practice nurse two days before a trip to receive the "necessary injections".

Poorly prepared business travellers run the risk of preventable ill health whilst abroad. This can take the form of physical or mental ill health, either of which will affect their ability to carry out the job effectively. Travellers who become unwell abroad can cost the sending company large amounts of money in medical bills or to cover the costs of repatriation. Time lost at work whilst abroad or on return is costly and further expense will be incurred if another employee has to be sent abroad to finish an incomplete job. For these reasons, it is wise for companies to take the time to prepare their employees for the trip—ultimately this will prove cost-effective, and the employees will be grateful for it.

Short hotel-based trips rarely cause too many problems, except perhaps loneliness, particularly if business travel is a common event. Loneliness can lead to overindulgence in alcohol and predispose to uncharacteristic behaviour, including sexual risk-taking with other travellers or commercial sex workers. Short term business trips are often arranged at the last minute, and may not allow adequate time for preparation, including rest, beforehand. Rest before a trip abroad is important, particularly if the journey is likely to be long. Lack of sleep can worsen jetlag, and tiredness plus jetlag is likely to affect efficiency.

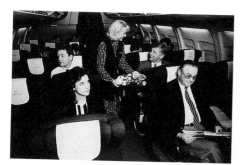

Longer business trips abroad can cause further problems. Cultural differences, language barriers, family problems at home, losing touch with head office, and a sense of isolation are more likely to occur. Infections and accidents are also more likely. Depending on the country, area to be visited, and the type of accommodation, additional vaccinations may be advised. Some business trips involve going to areas where there are few or very poor medical facilities and accommodation is basic. The purpose of this type of trip is often to develop an area. These projects can take many years and involve large numbers of employees going out repeatedly over a prolonged period. In those instances, it is particularly important for the employing authority to implement some sort of travel health programme.

Employees likely to be sent abroad at the last minute should be up to date with commonly recommended vaccines, such as polio, tetanus, typhoid, and hepatitis A. If there is the possibility of being sent to Africa or South America at short notice, it is wise to immunise against yellow fever, since it takes ten days for a certificate to be valid. For frequent travel to developing countries immunisation against hepatitis B should be considered. A full course of hepatitis B takes several months to complete.

Use of antimalarials can be complex for those travellers visiting many areas with different levels of risk. Long term use of antimalarials may involve rotating between different drugs and noncompliance and complacency is common in those who visit malarious areas often. This issue is too complex to generalise and each business traveller's needs should be considered individually.

Certain countries impose HIV entry restrictions on business or long term travellers and these are usually stipulated on visa requirements. This should be determined in advance since entry can be refused or "on the spot" testing carried out if requirements have not been fully met.

Many problems can be overcome by experience and sympathetic support from family, friends, and the company involved. Good insurance cover, including emergency repatriation, is important and reassuring. A medical contact at the destination is useful for those with pre-existing medical problems which could relapse. Frequent contact with family at home and the employing authority are also reassuring and can substantially reduce feelings of isolation and loneliness.

Beware of last minute assignments

Yellow fever certificates are valid only 10 days after a first dose

Jetlag can affect performance

Loneliness may be a problem

Package holiday makers

Package tours are extremely popular with tourists from many countries, including Britain. The main destinations from Britain for package tourists include Spain and its islands, Greece, Portugal and, increasingly, Turkey.

The whole idea of the package tour is that everything is organised via the travel agent and tour operator. This includes flights, transport from the airport, accommodation, sometimes meals and excursions, and there is usually a tour representative at the destination to help out with problems. Package tour destinations are assessed by the tour operators and graded accordingly. Theoretically, the traveller has a good idea of what to expect prior to leaving home and the package tour is often considered the safest type of travel. However, there are numerous hazards which can befall the tourist if care is not taken.

The idea that everything is organised by someone else can lead to a sense of carefree abandonment. This can lead to overindulgence in alcohol, promiscuity, uncharacteristic behaviour as the travellers "let their hair down", and reduced vigilance which can lead to accidents.

The most common health problems which affect package tourists can often be directly related to overindulgence of alcohol, such as diving accidents, road traffic accidents including falling off mopeds, and acquiring sexually transmitted diseases through casual sexual contacts. The problem of casual sex in tourists is particularly worrying since latest UK figures have shown that the fastest growing group of new HIV patients is heterosexuals who acquired the infection abroad. The recent trends in package tours to Africa, Asia, and sex tourist destinations will have an impact on these figures in years to come if this problem is not addressed.

Sunburn is common since many package tours are to sunny beach resorts. Weary holiday makers deprived of hot sunshine for many months often spend many hours sunbathing without adequate protection, despite the fact that this is now widely known to be dangerous.

The package tourist does not escape travellers' diarrhoea, and care with food and water hygiene is important, particularly for those countries with poor sanitation.

Whilst there are no additional vaccine recommendations for many European destinations, the increase in travel to Africa, Asia, and South America means that more package tourists are now being advised to be immunised. Many package tours are booked at the last minute, and this can lead to insufficient time for vaccines to become effective. Likewise, antimalarial chemoprophylaxis needs to be properly arranged.

Vaccinations may not be possible before last minute holidays

Take care over exposure to sun, accidents, and safe sex

Excessive alcohol drinking can cause problems

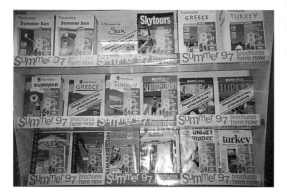

A great deal of faith is placed in tour operators to advise travellers on potential health hazards at the destination. The reality is that most tour operators are disinclined to give out this type of information for fear of putting potential travellers off and losing customers. In many instances no advice is given that vaccines and antimalarials may be needed or other health precautions necessary. The naive traveller may then embark on a trip to a high risk destination unprepared, and with a false sense of security.

Backpacking

Backpacking is the term used for self organised trips, where accommodation is not booked in advance and is usually basic and cheap, sometimes under canvas. Travel is generally by public transport or on foot. Trips are often prolonged and include visiting urban and rural areas. Visiting several different countries is common, and South East Asia is popular with British backpackers.

The very nature of backpacking increases exposure to a variety of health risks. Trekking on unexplored terrain or using public transport in poorly maintained, overcrowded vehicles on roads full of potholes, increases the risk of accidents. Backpackers are often young and this also increases the risk of accidents. If medical care, including blood transfusion is required, sterile blood and equipment may not be available. A comprehensive first aid kit (see chapter on first aid while abroad) including sterile needles and syringes is advised and comprehensive insurance is essential.

Backpackers do not usually follow traditional travel itineraries in main cities and tourist resorts, but like to go "off the beaten track". They are more likely to wander into areas of political unrest. Terrorists and bandits may be present and travellers should be aware of which areas to avoid.

Backpackers intending to mix with locals and visit isolated communities should respect local customs and values and should learn about them in advance. Travellers may need to adapt their dress code, to cover legs and shoulders for example. Unnecessary contact or conversation with local men by female travellers can be misinterpreted and should be avoided.

Clean water and safe food can be more difficult to obtain when away from main cities, especially when funds are limited. Most backpackers travel on a tight budget. Carrying a reliable method of water purification is important since bottled water can be expensive and is not always available (see chapter on preventing illness while abroad).

Budget accommodation and camping, particularly in rural areas, increases the risk of mosquito and other insect bites. Numerous infections can be transmitted by insect bites and care must be taken to avoid them. Backpackers should usually carry an impregnated mosquito net for protection, as portable nets are not readily available in many tropical countries. A course of emergency self treatment for malaria may be necessary, along with written instructions on how and when to use it (see chapter on malaria prevention).

Additional vaccines are often recommended for backpackers to certain countries, particularly for prolonged visits. This may include rabies vaccine if the traveller will be unable to obtain vaccine in the event of an animal bite. Hepatitis B vaccine should be considered since accidents may be more likely. Advice on avoiding hepatitis B and other blood borne infections such as hepatitis C and HIV should include avoiding drug injecting, acupuncture, body piercing and shaving from traditional barbers who re-use razors.

Backpackers who set out alone often meet with other similar travellers and drift into a commune lifestyle. This can reduce loneliness and alienation, but peer pressure can lead to activities such as drug taking and sexual promiscuity.

Though an exciting and challenging way to explore other countries and cultures, backpacking can be exhausting. Spare money for the odd night in comfort to recuperate is a good idea. Good comfortable shoes will make life easier. Buying cheap, appropriate clothing abroad can prevent setting out with an unreasonably heavy rucksack.

"Unusual" vaccinations are often necessary
Consider water sterilising equipment and a mosquito net
Be prepared for culture shock
Take extra money for emergencies

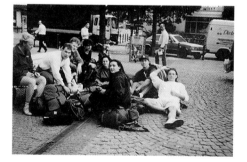

Expeditions

Take all recommended equipment

Beware of organisations that do not give advice on health precautions

Will leaders be carrying first aid supplies?

What arrangements are there for emergencies and repatriation?

Expeditions usually involve groups travelling together to areas that the average tourist would not consider exploring. This can mean visiting a remote area, travelling in difficult terrain, or seeking out people with unusual or different cultures. Expeditions often have a particular purpose—reaching the summit of Mount Everest, observing wildlife in the Amazon basin, or visting hilltribes in Tibet.

Expeditions are becoming more popular and can be well organised using well equipped, experienced guides, with participants well briefed in advance. Others are not so reliable. Research into details of what is offered by different agencies, perhaps paying particular attention to information on health issues, is worthwhile.

Expedition organisers should advise on:

- the proposed route in detail;
- modes of transport;
- accommodation;
- other facilities available;
- individual equipment required, and details of what is provided by the company;
- recommended suitable clothing;
- health recommendations prior to departure, including immunisation, chemoprophylaxis, emergency self treatments;
- insurance.

If there is no mention of preparation, provision of expert guides or issues related to health, a different organisation which gives more attention to safety should be considered.

Those with pre-exising illnesses and those who are unfit should pay particular attention to the physical effort involved and the availability of medical facilities. This is important both for the safety of the individual and the group as a whole since an ill prepared participant can burden other members of the group and jeopardise the entire party's safety.

Many of the health issues to consider are the same as for the backpacker—the risk of accidents, social etiquette, prevention of infections, additional vaccines, specialised equipment, supplies of self treatment for malaria and diarrhoea, comprehensive insurance cover. Sometimes there are medical or nursing personnel in the party, and certain health care equipment and medications may be available. Plans of action for emergencies and group insurance which covers repatriation may be supplied, but expedition travellers should not assume that all their individual needs will have been considered by the organisers. Group insurance may not cover those with a pre-existing illness. Insurance is only as good as the available facilities—repatriation from remote areas is not possible if the traveller has no contact with the outside world and cannot reach an airstrip; minor surgery cannot be performed if no one with experience is available.

When people who have never met before have to live, work, and get along with one another, in a close, often stressful environment, personality clashes or power struggles can occur. Inexperienced travellers can endanger themselves if they go off on their own, and jeopardise the safety of the others if the route has to be altered or the trip prolonged. Not everyone is suitable for expedition travel!

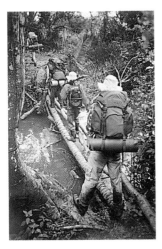

Tips for expedition travel

- Be prepared
- Respect the views of your leader and colleagues
- Be aware of your surroundings

Voluntary work overseas

Large numbers of volunteers offer their services abroad. The nature of their work is often diverse, and covers every kind of occupation imaginable. Time spent ranges from a few weeks to years (two years is the minimum commitment with Voluntary Services Overseas, one of the largest organisations). The destinations of volunteers include developing countries and areas of political unrest—common destinations recently for British volunteers include the former Yugoslavia, Romania, and Vietnam.

Some organisations which oversee relief workers and volunteers are extremely well organised, but others are less so. Inexperienced organisations do not always appreciate the importance of preparation relating to safety and health. It can be dangerous and costly to send ill prepared volunteers abroad into crisis situations, if they themselves become unwell, are unable to do the job intended, and then require repatriation.

Vaccinations, prevention of malaria, suitable equipment, prevention of HIV and sexually transmitted diseases, and food and water hygiene must all be considered. Many of the points already considered for the backpacker and expedition traveller apply.

Careful selection of volunteers is essential and organisations familiar with the problems associated with voluntary work and protracted overseas visits usually have rigorous selection procedures. Experienced professionals aim to select suitable candidates in an effort to avoid problems for the individual, other volunteers, and the hosts.

While volunteers are often sent to areas where poverty and disease are commonplace and they may have to cope with situations they previously could not have imagined, voluntary work can be immensely satisfying and life-enriching, and many choose to extend their stay.

"Culture shock" on return home is a very real problem. Many have given up jobs and homes and their contact with family and friends may have been irregular. The new "family" and friends have been local people and other volunteers and the process of saying "goodbye" has to start all over again as the return date approaches. It can be difficult to settle back into the previous lifestyle where materialism and "self sufficiency" (selfishness) are unrecognised norms. Keeping in contact with other volunteers and friends in the host country can ease this sense of alienation, which is often not anticipated.

- Many will be young and it will be the first trip abroad
- Select postings carefully—they are usually for less than 2 years
- There may be little time to learn the local language
- Facilities are often primitive
- Volunteers take skills but the learning is "both ways"

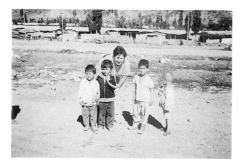

The long term expatriate

Preparation and health considerations for long term or indefinite periods abroad can become very complex, particularly when whole families are involved. Whenever possible, ample time should be allowed and preparation not rushed. A brief visit to the proposed destination in advance can help reduce fear of the unknown. Finding out about local conditions and medical facilities in advance can affect recommendations prior to departure. Contact with the British embassy may be useful, particularly in areas with political unrest. If possible, contact with other expatriates should be made as their advice can be invaluable.

Vaccinations, prevention of malaria (if appropriate), first aid equipment, food and water hygiene, how to avoid diseases for which there are no vaccines such as HIV infection, and what to do in an emergency all need careful consideration, particularly for those going to areas with basic or remote medical facilities.

Many of the points already outlined for other groups of travellers are relevant, but even more so since the time at risk will be prolonged.

Children and young infants may not have completed (or even started) primary immunisations before the departure date and courses started in Britain may require boosters at the destination. Special advice on malaria prevention should include the possible need for emergency self treatments and whether chemoprophylaxis should be taken indefinitely. Eye and dental check ups before departure help avoid the problem of having to locate a dentist or optician soon after arrival in the host country. Women of child bearing age should consider the implications of pregnancy especially if going to live in areas with minimal facilities. Those with a pre-existing illness should seek advice from their doctor before departure.

The reason for moving abroad can have an impact on adaptation to new circumstances of those involved. Those who move as a planned event may have fewer problems than those who feel that they "had no choice". Many families move for better employment opportunities of one partner, usually the husband. As a result the roles of the entire family can change dramatically, for example the wife gives up work completely, the children move to a different education system. Living with people of another culture, learning a new language, and leaving family and friends are challenges which raise difficulties. Initial

---

- Go out of your way to make new friends
- Learn the local language
- Consider schooling for children
- What about possible pregnancy?
- Check in advance about local medical facilities

developmental "regression" in children undergoing such changes is not uncommon and patience and understanding is required from the parents.

Homesickness often develops after a few months, when the initial excitement of the new environment begins to wear off and the realisation that the move is not short term sinks in. Trips home at this stage are not always a good idea but frequent contact with people at home is usually helpful. Letters and telephone calls take on a new importance which can be impressed on those at home.

Making new friends and being sensitive rather than critical to cultural differences will assist the settling in process. Trying to make everything the same as at home is likely to lead to frustrated disappointment.

Living and working abroad and raising a family in a different environment poses many challenges but most will not regret the experience.

Not every one **can** adapt. Professional screening before such moves may identify some of those who are not suitable and allow alternative destinations or dates of departure to be considered.

IMMUNISATION

Some basic principles of immunisation

<table>
<tr><td>

Immunisation

Those receiving vaccines are usually fit but often anxious

Faints are more likely in those with hypoglycaemia (e.g. after no breakfast)

Anaphylaxis is very rare but facilities must be available in case it occurs

Prescribing vaccines needs the same considerations as when using other medications, e.g. assessing risk/benefit, dose, contraindications, possible side effects, cost

</td></tr>
</table>

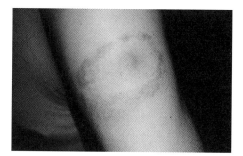

All vaccines have potential for causing side effects—a sore arm after diptheria immunisation. Benefits should outweigh any risks.

Active immunisation is when the body's own immune system is stimulated by administering:

- *live attenuated organisms* (for example, BCG, oral poliomyelitis, yellow fever, measles, mumps, rubella);
- *inactivated organisms* (for example, rabies, Japanese B encephalitis, hepatitis A);
- *toxoids* (for example, diphtheria, tetanus);
- *components of organisms* such as capsular polysaccharides or subunits (for example, typhoid Vi, meningococcal, pneumococcal);
- *genetically engineered* viral products (for example, hepatitis B).

Advantages of active vaccination are that long term immunity is usually achieved, especially with live vaccines. A disadvantage is that immunity is not gained immediately. *Combined active vaccines* are becoming more common but vaccines should not be "mixed" in the surgery.

Passive immunisation involves the administration of immunoglobulin containing appropriate antibodies acquired from blood donations. Immunity is gained immediately but is short-lived. Sometimes normal pooled immunoglobulin contains sufficient antibodies to be protective (against hepatitis A, for example) but specific immunoglobulin may need to be prepared, for example, by collecting blood from actively immunised donors as in hepatitis B or rabies.

Primary courses consist of one or more doses. There is an interval before protective immunity is gained; this is usually at least 2 weeks, often longer. Usually intervals can be prolonged without loss of protection but doses given too close together may not give the desired maximum response.

Boosters are given at intervals varying with the vaccine.

Interactions: if immunoglobulin is given with or before a live vaccine the response to the latter may be suboptimal. Live vaccines should be given at the same time or separated by 3 weeks to avoid a suboptimal response from the later vaccination due to "interference".

Routes of administration may be intra-muscular, subcutaneous or intra-dermal and vary with the specific vaccines. This should always be checked. For example giving diphtheria vaccine intra-dermally instead of deep subcutaneously can result in a very sore arm, but equally giving BCG subcutaneously can result in an abcess at the site of the injection.

Contraindications must always be checked with the manufacturer's literature and often include, for example, fever, previous reactions, pregnancy, immunocompromise (for example, from medications), and pregnancy. As well as sometimes being a contraindication to live vaccines, immunocompromise (including HIV infection) may result in a poor immune response.

Probable and confirmed adverse reactions must always be carefully assessed, recorded in the patient's notes and reported to both the Committee on Safety of Medicines and the manufacturers. Anaphylaxis and angioneurotic oedema, for example, are contraindications to further doses of the same vaccine.

Storage and reconstitution instructions must be carefully followed. Some vaccines may be destroyed by heat although many are stable for quite long periods at room temperature. Others are inactivated by freezing. When vaccines have to be reconstituted they may then only be active for a few hours.

Records: when vaccines have been administered records should ideally be kept both by the surgery and by the patient (for example in booklets for patients to keep with their passport). When vaccines are administered by dedicated NHS or private travel clinics the patient's general practitioner should also be informed.

Assessing the risk

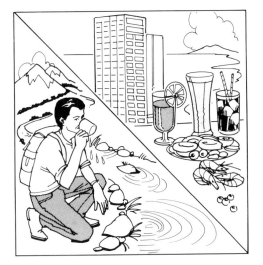

Travellers are particularly liable to contract infections because they are exposed to pathogens that are absent or uncommon in their country of residence. Furthermore, contact with these organisms is increased through food and water contamination, biting arthropods, and increased human contact of varying intimacy. When planning a vaccination schedule, the likelihood of the individual traveller acquiring a particular disease should be assessed. This should take into account the following.

● *Prevalence of disease at the destination.* Many diseases causing illness in travellers originate in the tropics. Travel to more temperate areas of the world, such as North America, Canada, Australia, New Zealand, Western Europe, and Japan, poses few incremental risks.
● *Duration of stay.* Longer stays allow a greater opportunity for infection to occur. Some infections may also have a varying seasonal risk.
● *Occupation.* Some activities entail risk from specific infections, for example midwives and veterinarians.
● *Standard of hygiene.* Purity of local water and food supplies may be poor. The local population may have a higher prevalence of carriers of pathogens such as *Salmonella typhi*. Personal hygiene may be difficult to achieve in countries with a shortage of water for washing.
● *Lifestyle and mode of travel.* An overland traveller in the tropics eating and drinking local food and water is clearly at more risk of disease than one staying for a week in a good hotel in Europe. In general, inexperience, travel within rural areas, using public transport, mixing closely with local people, eating out, and sexual promiscuity place the traveller at higher risk of disease.

Other factors that need to be considered before a schedule for immunisation can be drawn up include the individual's previous vaccination and travel history, medical history, and any current illnesses, whether they are pregnant or planning on becoming pregnant, are taking medications, have certain allergies or are immunocompromised. Remember that only a very small percentage of travel related illness is preventable with vaccines and no vaccine is 100% effective. Travellers need a broader perspective than discovering which "jabs" are required and the general health measures to prevent illness whilst abroad, described in subsequent chapters, should be emphasised during the travel consultation.

Immunisation may conveniently be considered under the following headings of *compulsory*, where evidence of vaccination is a prerequisite for entry into a country, *commonly recommended* and *sometimes recommended*.

Compulsory

Yellow fever

Yellow fever is caused by a virus that circulates enzootically in certain tropical forested areas of Africa and South America. It mainly infects monkeys but if man enters these areas the virus may be transmitted to him by mosquitoes whose normal hosts are these monkeys. This is "jungle" yellow fever. It occurs haphazardly and is clearly related to man's habits. If, after originating from an enzootic source, the virus begins to circulate between man and his own mosquitoes, primarily *Aedes aegypti*, epidemics of "urban" yellow fever result.

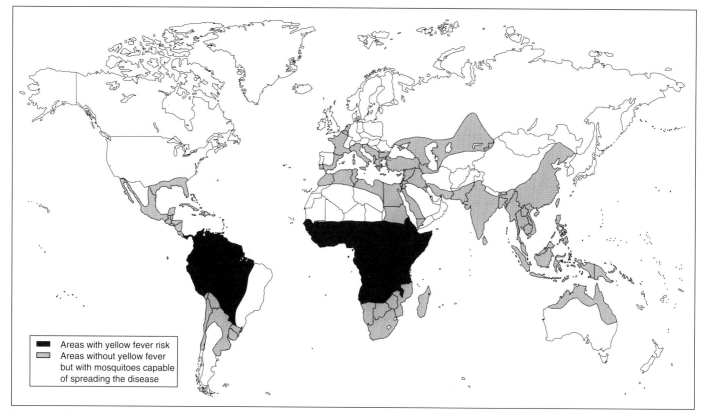

Adapted with permission from *International travel and health. Vaccination requirements and health advice 1996*. Geneva: WHO, 1996.

Immunisation protects the individual and is effective in preventing spread of the virus to countries where *A aegypti* is prevalent but the disease is absent. Such countries request a certificate of vaccination from travellers coming from areas where yellow fever infections occur. Countries where the disease is present may also require immunisation of travellers entering from all countries, or else if entering from other "infected areas". A map of zones where yellow fever is endemic (enzootic) is shown. Lists of countries' requirements are readily available (see chapter on information sources and wall chart).

Immunisation is clearly not indicated when travelling outside the enzootic zones. Within the zones, if it is not compulsory it is not always necessary. For instance, in the absence of an epidemic of yellow fever a business trip within the confines of Nairobi would be perfectly safe. Nevertheless, local and current knowledge of cases is required for such decisions to be made, so in practice immunisation is usually recommended to all travellers to these areas.

Immunisation is undertaken only at recognised yellow fever vaccination centres registered with the World Health Organisation so that internationally valid certificates can be issued. Those wishing to register as a yellow fever centre should contact the Department of Health, or in Scotland, the Scottish Office Home and Health Department.

Yellow fever vaccine (Evans Medical)

- Live attenuated virus—17D strain
- Single 0·5 ml dose given subcutaneously
- Boost every 10 years
- Side effects—occasionally mild headache, myalgia, low-grade fever, local reactions. Very rarely encephalitis has occurred in very young infants
- Contraindications—<9 months old, pregnant, immunosuppressed, severe egg hypersensitivity, acute febrile illness, severe reaction to a previous dose
- Comment—certificate valid after 10 days for 10 years

Commonly recommended

Typhim Vi vaccine (Pasteur Merieux)

- Vi capsular polysaccharide antigen of *Salmonella typhi*
- Single 0·5 ml dose given deep subcutaneously or intramuscularly
- Boost every 3 years
- Side effects—occasionally mild local reactions
- Contraindications—pregnancy (unless the risk of infection is substantial), acute febrile illness, severe reaction to a previous dose
- Comment—response may be less in children <18 months

Typhoid fever

Spread of typhoid fever is usually faecal-oral. The risk of infection is increased in areas of high carriage rates and poor hygiene. The risk is not significantly increased for the traveller from Britain to areas with similar public health standards—namely, Europe, the United States of America, Canada, Australia, New Zealand, and Japan. Outside these areas the risks reflect not only local hygiene and carriage rates but also lifestyle. Travelling or living rough, living in rural areas, or "eating out" makes faecal-oral transmission of any pathogen more likely. The risks are therefore small for the air traveller with full board at a reputable hotel. On the other hand, overland travel to Australia would

---

Oral typhoid vaccine (Evans Medical)

Attenuated Ty 21a strain of *Salmonella typhi*
- 1 capsule orally on days 1, 3, and 5
- Boost 1–3 yearly repeating 3 dose course
- Side effects—occasionally nausea, vomiting, diarrhoea, rash
- Contraindications—pregnancy, immunocompromised individuals and those taking antibiotics, sulphonamides or mefloquine
- Comment—not for use in children <6 years. Separate from oral polio by at least 2 weeks

---

Havrix monodose/Junior Havrix monodose (SmithKline Beecham)

- Formaldehyde inactivated hepatitis A virus
- Adults—single 1 ml dose of Havrix given intramuscularly protects for up to a year
- Children <16 years—single 0.5 ml dose of Junior Havrix given intramuscularly protects for up to a year
- Boost using single dose at 6–12 months to confer 10 years immunity
- Side effects—occasionally mild local reactions. Rarely fever, malaise, headache, GI upset.
- Contraindications—same as for other inactivated vaccines
- Comment—protects 10–14 days after primary dose

Avaxim (Pasteur Merieux)

- Formaldehyde inactivated hepatitis A virus
- Single 0.5 ml dose given intramuscularly protects for at least 6 months
- Boost using single dose at 6 months to protect for up to 10 years
- Side effects—occasionally local pain, myalgia, headache, GI upset, and fever. Rarely local erythema
- Contraindications—same as for other inactivated vaccines
- Comment—only for those aged >16 years. No paediatric preparation available as yet

---

Oral poliomyelitis vaccine (Sabin)

- Live attenuated vaccine—three serotypes
- 3 drops orally given 3 times at monthly intervals
- Boost every 10 years with 3 drops
- Side effects—rarely cases of vaccine-associated polio are reported
- Contraindications—acute or febrile illness, vomiting or diarrhoea, immunosuppression, pregnancy
- Comment—try to give at the same time as other live vaccines or else separate by 3 weeks

---

be a clear indication for immunisation. Between these extremes there are many circumstances for which risks cannot be precisely defined, where, for example, immunisation may be advisable for those whose lifestyle or length of stay increases the risk of exposure and during local outbreaks.

Only monovalent typhoid vaccine is now produced because of the lack of efficacy and the side effects associated with the paratyphoid A and B components of TAB vaccine. The traditional inactivated vaccine (Evans) is abut 70–90% effective but is renowned for causing unpleasant side effects, although these can be reduced by administering the vaccine intradermally. This vaccine is currently unavailable in the UK and its relicensing is being reviewed.

Oral live attenuated and Vi capsular polysaccharide vaccines are now available in Britain. The oral vaccine requires three doses for a primary course, giving up to 70% protection for up to three years and has no recognised serious adverse reactions. It must be stored in a refrigerator and the capsules should be swallowed whole, one hour before a meal, with a cold or lukewarm drink—thus efficacy is very much related to patient compliance. The USA datasheet for this vaccine advises taking four doses to confer five years immunity, a more preferable option to that currently advised in the UK. The Vi capsular polysaccharide vaccine requires only one dose for a primary course to give similar protection to the traditional vaccine but with substantially fewer side effects.

Hepatitis A

Hepatitis A virus is endemic worldwide and spread by the faecal-oral route; protection from symptomatic infection can be provided by active vaccination or from immunoglobulin. The virus circulates freely in our own population, however, and many travellers will be immune already. For instance, about half those over 50 years old in Scotland have hepatitis A antibodies, although prevalence is lower in England and Wales, and among those from higher socioeconomic backgrounds.

Before vaccination is given to those with a history of jaundice, with probable exposure, or over the age of around 40 years, it is reasonable to check for the presence of hepatitis A antibody. When IgG is present the person is immune for life and vaccination is unnecessary.

Active vaccination against hepatitis A is available and should be considered for travellers to areas of moderate or high endemicity. Both vaccines available in the UK are highly immunogenic, conferring long-term immunity of up to 10 years after two doses. Passive immunisation using human normal immunoglobulin (HNIG) is an alternative, although this offers only short term protection of between 2 and 6 months, depending on the dose administered. In adults, 250 mg of HNIG given intramuscularly will protect for 2 months, 500 mg for 4 months and 750 mg for 6 months. Children older than 10 years can be given roughly half these doses. HNIG gives immediate protection, useful for the traveller who attends too late for active vaccination. It may be administered at the same time as vaccine although this may lessen the duration of protection. The Blood Transfusion Service in Scotland will supply HNIG for use in travellers. Elsewhere in the UK it is only available commercially.

Poliomyelitis

Polio viruses are usually spread faecal–orally, but in the acute phase may also be spread by droplets from the nasopharynx. Poliomyelitis remains endemic in many countries with a low level of public hygiene. Live, oral poliomyelitis vaccine is normally used in Britain, but inactivated polio vaccine is available if oral vaccine is contraindicated, as in pregnancy, the immunocompromised, or if the vaccine has to be given at the same time as immunoglobulin. The inactivated vaccine is unlicensed in the UK and requires to be ordered on a named-patient basis from Farillon (01708 379000) or through the community pharmacy.

Tetanus vaccine (T) (Evans)

- Formaldehyde inactivated tetanus toxin
- 3 × 0·5 ml dose given deep subcutaneously or intramuscularly at monthly intervals
- Boost 10 yearly with single dose
- Side effects—local reactions fairly common
- Contraindications—same as for other inactivated vaccines
- Comment—plain tetanus vaccine (without adjuvant) is no longer available

---

Tetanus

As the source of tetanus spores is environmental, herd immunity is irrelevant and immunisation is solely for the benefit of the individual. It is as firmly recommended for life in Britain as for travel abroad. Recent studies suggest one in eight of the population are not adequately protected.

There are various preparations of tetanus vaccine available in the UK. Tetanus is combined with diphtheria and pertussis (DPT) or with diphtheria alone (DT) for use in children up to 10 years, as a component of the British childhood immunisation programme. Single antigen tetanus vaccine (T) can be used in all age groups and when combined with a low dose preparation of diphtheria toxoid (Td) is suitable for adults and children older than 10 years.

Remember, when treating serious, potentially contaminated wounds, tetanus immunoglobulin should be used in conjunction with tetanus toxoid.

Sometimes recommended

BCG

Tuberculosis is usually spread via respiratory droplets, although it may be transmitted through ingestion of unpasteurised infected milk. It can affect any organ of the body but most commonly affects the lungs or lymph nodes.

In Britain BCG proved effective in reducing both the incidence and severity of tuberculosis in schoolchildren. National policy is to recommend immunisation to all tuberculin-negative 11–13 year olds and to immunise younger children only if there is a family history or exposure risk. If children or non-vaccinated adults are to live in areas of increased risk, especially Africa, Asia, and south or central America, immunisation of those whose skin test results are negative should be recommended.

A single dose of 0·1 ml BCG (0·05 ml for infants <3 months) should be given intradermally over the insertion of the left deltoid. Normally a small blister appears at the site which may take several weeks to heal, leaving a characteristic scar. Large ulcers and abscesses following BCG administration are usually as a result of faulty immunisation technique (giving the injection too deeply) or because the individual is already sensitive to tuberculoprotein. It can be given from birth. Tuberculosis is becoming more common worldwide and is often an opportunistic infection in AIDS.

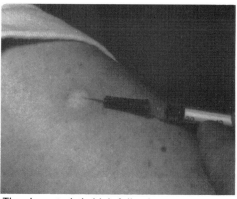

The characteristic bleb following administration of BCG.

Diphtheria

Diphtheria is an acute upper respiratory tract infection spread by aerosol inhalation of infected droplets. From 1986 to 1991, 13 cases of diphtheria were reported in Britain. Most were traced to an imported source, usually an asymptomatic carrier. Risk of infection is greater when overcrowding and low levels of vaccine uptake co-exist, as is witnessed in Africa, Asia, and Central and South America. When the diphtheria organism circulates freely most adults are immune, but with routine childhood immunisation interrupting transmission of the organism, increasing numbers of adults are susceptible. Most morbidity and mortality occurs in children, who should be immunised as nationally recommended. A recent death occurred in a teenager travelling from Britain to Pakistan who had not been previously immunised. Adult travellers at high risk of infection are those in contact with children in endemic areas—for example, health workers and teachers. There has been an increase in cases from the Russian Federation and Ukraine due to recent population movement, declining childhood immunisation uptake, and waning immunity in the adult population. Booster doses of diphtheria toxoid should be given every 10 years to those at risk. Schick testing before booster immunisations is unnecessary if the low dose preparation of the vaccine is used. If no low dose preparation is available, 0·1 ml of the single antigen diphtheria vaccine may be given deep subcutaneously or intramuscularly.

Diphtheria vaccines

Children < 10 years
- Diphtheria, pertussis, tetanus vaccine (DPT)
- Diphtheria, tetanus vaccine (DT)
- Single antigen diphtheria vaccine (D)

Adults and children > 10 years
- Low dose diphtheria vaccine (d)
- Tetanus combined with low dose diphtheria vaccine (Td)

- Three doses of a suitable preparation should be given at monthly intervals for primary immunisation. Children should receive school entry and school leaving booster doses. Adults require 10 yearly boosters if at risk

---

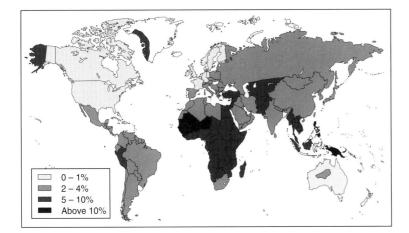

World distribution of HBsAg carriage. The two areas of higher incidence in Australasia represent Aboriginal (Central Australia) and Maori (New Zealand) populations.

Legend:
- 0 – 1%
- 2 – 4%
- 5 – 10%
- Above 10%

Hepatitis B

Hepatitis B vaccine should be recommended for groups such as medical, nursing, and laboratory staff planning to work among populations with high carriage rates of HBsAg. It can also be considered for those planning to live long term in such regions. There is evidence that children in areas of high hepatitis B carriage commonly contract the infection after starting school. Infant vaccination is now being recommended worldwide by the World Health Organisation as a means of preventing perinatal transmission of a carrier state.

Three doses are normally given, the second and third after one and six months. An accelerated schedule involves three doses at 0, one, and two months with a booster after one year. Vaccination must be given intramuscularly, in the deltoid area or, in children and infants, in the anterolateral area of the thigh. A half dose is given to children under 12 years and immunocompromised patients may respond only to a double dose or not at all. About 5% of recipients do not develop antibodies—whether this means they are unprotected is unclear.

Meningococcal vaccine (Pasteur Merieux, SmithKline Beecham)

- A and C polysaccharide vaccine
- Single dose of 0·5 ml given deep subcutaneously or intramuscularly
- Boost with a single dose after 3–5 years
- Side effects—mild local reactions
- Contraindications—not recommended <2 months of age
- Comments—immune response is poor in children <18 months. A certificate of vaccination is required of all visitors to the Haj in Saudi Arabia

Meningococcal A and C

Regular epidemics of meningococcal A disease develop in the "meningitis belt" of Africa—the countries bordering the southern Sahara and southern end of the Nile valley extending as far south as Zambia and Malawi. The outbreaks are usually in the hot dry season in the first six months of the year. It is spread through close person to person contact (for example, within families, schools, dormitories), hence the risk is usually small for organised "package" tourists. Sporadic outbreaks of type A have been seen in India, Brazil, Nepal, Mongolia, and Saudi Arabia. Vaccine is available only against groups A and C, and is recommended for travel to areas where outbreaks are present and for prolonged visits to the meningitis belt. There have been several small outbreaks of meningococcal infection in recent years in tourist resorts in the Spanish islands. This is not surprising when large numbers of people are living in close proximity. None of these outbreaks has consistently been due to any particular serotype and vaccination has not been recommended.

Rabies vaccine (Pasteur Merieux)

- Inactivated human diploid cell vaccine
- 1 ml subcutaneously on days 0, 7, and 28 or 0·1 ml intradermally at same intervals)
- Boost 2–3 yearly with single dose
- Side effects—mainly local reactions
- Contraindications—same as for other inactivated vaccines
- Comment—can be prescribed under the NHS for those at occupational risk of infection, e.g. veterinarians

Rabies

Rabies is spread via a bite or scratch from an infected animal, usually a dog, but any warm blooded mammal may transmit the infection. The virus attacks the central nervous system and rabies is invariably fatal once symptoms have developed.

Human diploid cell vaccine (the only inactivated rabies vaccine available in Britain) is effective and has few side effects. Pre-exposure prophylaxis should be recommended for high risk groups such as veterinarians working in areas enzootic for rabies, and for those staying in these areas who will be more than a day's journey away from a source of post-exposure vaccination. Pre-exposure prophylaxis is usually given by the intramuscular route in Britain. This route should be used if chloroquine is being taken concurrently as chloroquine may lower the immune response. It has also been successfully given intradermally and this is the usual route of administration in the United States although this route is not covered by the UK data sheet. Post-exposure prophylaxis with human diploid cell vaccine is also effective, but there have been two reports of rabies developing after the use of post-exposure courses of vaccine in addition to rabies specific hyperimmunoglobulin. (See First Aid chapter for treatment of suspect

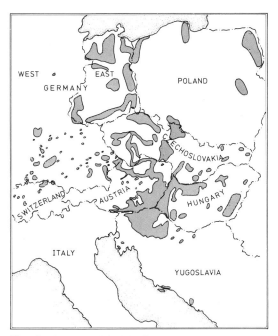

The distribution of TBE in Europe.

Japanese B encephalitis vaccine (Biken, Green Cross)

- Formaldehyde inactivated whole cell vaccine
- 3 × 1 ml dose given deep subcutaneously on days 0, 7–14 and 30 (3 × 0·5 ml for children <3 years)
- Two doses given 1–4 weeks apart will confer short term immunity of about 3 months
- Boost 2 yearly with a single dose
- Side effects—small risk of urticaria and angioedema developing up to 2 weeks after vaccination
- Contraindications—previous anaphylaxis
- Comment—only use in children <1 year if exposure to infection is unavoidable. JE vaccine is available only on named patient basis in UK

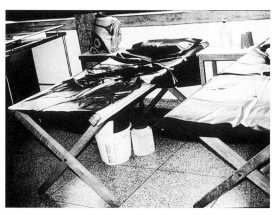

An example of a "cholera bed" showing a plastic sheet with bucket to collect and measure faecal fluid.

---

bites.) In both patients vaccine was given in the gluteal region instead of the recommended deltoid area. Despite these failures, post-exposure use of the vaccine is still highly effective and the chance of receiving a rabid bite is slim. A pre-exposure course should always be followed by post-exposure boosters as soon as possible after a suspect bite.

Tick borne encephalitis

Tick borne encephalitis is caused by a flavivirus transmitted by the bite of an infected tick. Its distribution is mainly in low forested areas in parts of Scandinavia, the Commonwealth of Independent States (formerly USSR), central Europe, particularly Austria, Czechoslovakia, West Germany, and northern areas of the former Yugoslavia. The forests are usually deciduous with heavy undergrowth. Those normally at risk are foresters and those clearing such areas, but contact occurs with recreational use, such as camping and walking. Most illness occurs in late spring and early summer. Tick bites are best avoided by limiting contact with long grass, wearing clothing to cover most of the skin surface (socks outside trousers), and using insect repellents on outer clothes and socks. Where prolonged contact is unavoidable a killed vaccine is available from Immuno Ltd for named patients only. Two doses are necessary 2–12 weeks apart to confer immunity for up to one year, with a booster dose at 9–12 months protecting for 3 years. Hyperimmune–globulin is available from hospital emergency departments in "at risk" areas on the continent of Europe for use within four days of a tick bite, and from Immuno Ltd in Britain.

Japanese B encephalitis

This arboviral infection is transmitted by the bite of an infected culicine mosquito that normally breeds in rice paddies. The main host is probably the pig but other animals and some birds may also be affected. The disease is endemic throughout Asia and some Pacific islands, and epidemics may develop wherever these factors coexist, especially during the monsoon—for example, in northern Thailand, north east India, and eastern Nepal.

The vaccine is indicated for those staying in these areas for long periods and for those not likely to be able to avoid mosquito bites (for example, if staying in poorer quality accommodation). Although rare in travellers, the disease can be severe, particularly in children (up to 30% mortality in symptomatic cases), and this vaccine is becoming more widely used. Rashes can occur, particularly after the first dose.

Cholera

In 1973 the World Health Organisation, recognising that immunisation cannot stop the spread of cholera among countries, deleted from the International Health Regulations the requirement of cholera immunisation as a condition of admission to any country. No country now officially requires certificates from travellers entering from an infected area, and the World Health Organisation no longer supplies them. Occasionally they are still asked for at international borders in remote areas where a government's requirements may not always be adhered to. Cholera vaccine is no longer available in the UK.

A survey of reported cholera in travellers indicated that the risks of infection are extremely low, even allowing for underreporting and illness occurring while in the country visited. Cholera immunisation gives only poor, short-lived protection. Most at risk are those using untreated drinking water in sub-Saharan Africa, tropical Asia, and more recently south and central America. Prevention depends upon food and particularly water hygiene.

Plague

Plague is an infection of wild rodents and is transmitted by fleas. It exists in many areas of Africa, Asia, and the Americas, though most reported human cases in 1994 were infected in India, Myanmar, Vietnam, Zaire, and Madagascar. The risk to the traveller is from the bite of an infected flea and is low. Routine immunisation is not recommended. In enzootic areas contact with rodents should be discouraged by preventing their access to food and waste, avoiding dead

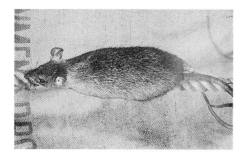

rodents and rodent burrows. Fleas can be discouraged by insect repellents. When prolonged stay in a rural enzootic area is expected and avoidance of rodents impracticable—for example, during wars or after disasters—an inactivated vaccine is available. Two doses are necessary 4 to 12 weeks apart with subsequent boosters every six months. Transport of the vaccine is difficult because of "cold chain" requirements, and it is therefore expensive, and currently has to be imported into Britain for named patients only (contact Bayer UK Ltd). Diagnosed early, plague is normally curable with tetracyclines, chloramphenicol or streptomycin.

New vaccines

A number of new vaccines are currently under development or being considered. These include vaccines against dengue and meningococcal group B infection, oral vaccines against cholera and *E. coli* enteritis (a common cause of traveller's diarrhoea). A combined vaccine against hepatitis A and B has just been released.

The role of the travel clinic

> **Main considerations of setting up a travel clinic**
>
> - Providing a suitable environment
> - Utilising staff with appropriate education
> - Allocating responsibilities
> - Drawing up practice protocols
> - Storing and ordering vaccines
> - Administering vaccines
> - Becoming a designated yellow fever vaccinating centre
> - Preparing for anaphylaxis
> - Documentation
> - Prescribing responsibilities
> - Accessing reliable and up-to-date reference sources
> - Allocating clinic time
> - Providing commodities other than vaccines
> - Providing literature
> - Generating income
> - Audit

In recent years there has been an increase in the number of designated travel clinics in response to ever increasing demands from the general public. Travel clinics can be found in general practices, health centres, occupational health departments, and in association with travel agents.

Preparatory research into the need and likely competition for such a service is necessary, since not all areas have sufficient demand.

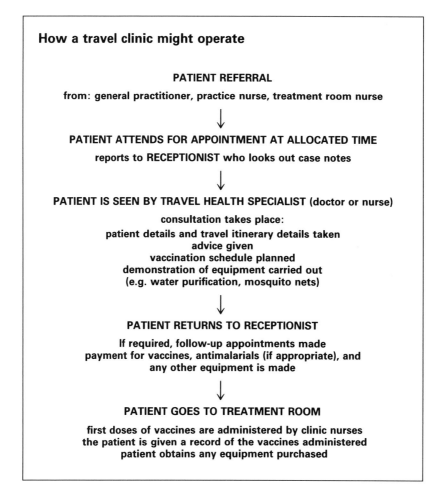

> **How a travel clinic might operate**
>
> **PATIENT REFERRAL**
> from: general practitioner, practice nurse, treatment room nurse
>
> ↓
>
> **PATIENT ATTENDS FOR APPOINTMENT AT ALLOCATED TIME**
> reports to RECEPTIONIST who looks out case notes
>
> ↓
>
> **PATIENT IS SEEN BY TRAVEL HEALTH SPECIALIST (doctor or nurse)**
> consultation takes place:
> patient details and travel itinerary details taken
> advice given
> vaccination schedule planned
> demonstration of equipment carried out
> (e.g. water purification, mosquito nets)
>
> ↓
>
> **PATIENT RETURNS TO RECEPTIONIST**
> If required, follow-up appointments made
> payment for vaccines, antimalarials (if appropriate), and
> any other equipment is made
>
> ↓
>
> **PATIENT GOES TO TREATMENT ROOM**
> first doses of vaccines are administered by clinic nurses
> the patient is given a record of the vaccines administered
> patient obtains any equipment purchased

Arranging a schedule

- Check intervals for primary courses
- Remember yellow fever certificate is valid only after 10 days
- Give live vaccines together if possible, or three weeks apart
- Give immunoglobulin just before departure
- The only reason for separating inactivated vaccines is for comfort of the patients

Remember to find out:

Previous vaccination history
Country(ies) to be visited
Likely lifestyle and accommodation
Any occupational risk
Duration of stay
Date of departure

Is the traveller:

Taking any medication?
Suffering from any existing illness?
Allergic to any relevant drugs or eggs?
Pregnant or likely soon to become so?

Interactions between vaccines

- Oral poliomyelitis vaccine should be given three weeks before, or three months after, immunoglobulin to give maximum response
- Live virus vaccines should be given either simultaneously, or at least three weeks apart, to avoid the response to the second vaccine being lowered by interferon produced in response to the first
- All the inactivated vaccines can be given in any combination with any other vaccine.

Live attenuated vaccines:

BCG (against tuberculosis)
Measles
Mumps
Poliomyelitis (oral)
Rubella
Typhoid (oral)
Yellow fever

Non-live vaccines:

Cholera	Meningococcal
Diphtheria (toxoid)	Pertussis
Haemophilus	Pneumococcal
influenzae (HIB)	Poliomyelitis
Hepatitis A	(injectable)
Hepatitis B	Rabies
Influenza	Tetanus (toxoid)
Japanese B	Tick borne encephalitis
encephalitis	Typhoid (injectable)

MALARIA PREVENTION

Why is there concern?

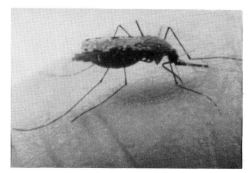

The female anophilene mosquito preparing to feed.

Malaria is widespread in tropical and subtropical areas of the world and is spread by the bite of a female anopheline mosquito that has been infected by the malaria parasite.

During the 1960s control measures in many areas seemed to be bringing malaria under control. A resurgence has occurred, however, particularly in the Indian subcontinent, parts of South America, and Africa. Reasons for this include the cost of maintaining control programmes, lack of enthusiasm for preventive measures when the disease is becoming uncommon, the developing resistance of mosquitoes to insecticides, and drug resistance of the parasites themselves.

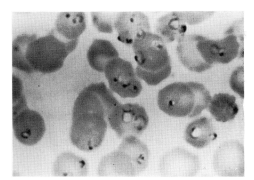

Red blood cells heavily infected with *P. falciparum* trophozoites.

The increasing mobility of the population, especially through air travel, brings a further hazard as travellers may be bitten by mosquitoes at airports en route as well as in the countries where they stay. The speed of travel means that initial symptoms may occur in a country and in a context where the disease will not be immediately considered. Mosquitoes may even be brought in aeroplanes to non-endemic areas and infect, for example, airport staff or travellers' relatives. Infection also occurs through blood transfusion (cold storage does not destroy the parasites) and the sharing of needles by intravenous drug misusers.

The most immediately life threatening form of malaria is caused by *Plasmodium falciparum*. Many more people are now travelling to Africa from Britain and there were approximately 1000 imported cases of falciparum malaria in 1996 compared with 200 in 1976. Prevention is primarily aimed at this parasite. Nevertheless, the same advice is given to those likely to be exposed to the less dangerous *P vivax*, *P malariae*, and *P ovale*, partly to prevent an unpleasant illness but also because *P falciparum* infection can never be presumed to be absent in any malarious area.

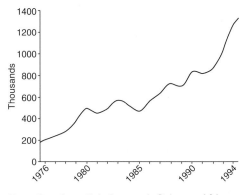

Travellers from Britain to sub-Saharan Africa at risk of falciparum malaria.

There is no immediate prospect of an effective vaccine, so avoiding mosquito bites and, often, the use of prophylactic tablets are both necessary. Some find taking preventative medicines difficult or even distasteful, but if appropriate tablets are being taken falciparum malaria can usually be prevented. Prompt and appropriate treatment is a third line of defence—of increasing importance in areas of resistance of *P falciparum* to the usual prophylactic drugs.

P vivax and *P ovale* have persistent liver forms and illness may result up to a year or more after exposure even if prophylaxis has been taken "correctly". When this occurs treatment with primaquine to destroy these liver forms may be required.

Be aware of the risk and take precautions

Remember

- Be aware of the risk of malaria
- Wear long trousers, long sleeves, dresses, and socks
- Use insect repellents on exposed skin
- Use insect repellents also on clothing around ankles, wrists, and collar
- Use a mosquito net impregnated with an insecticide
- Use insecticide spray in your room if necessary
- Take your anti-malaria tablets regularly

Prophylactic drugs available in Britain

Chloroquine
Formulation:
  150 mg of base
Adult prophylactic dose:
  Two tablets weekly

Proguanil
Formulation:
  100 mg
Adult prophylactic dose:
  Two tablets daily

Mefloquine
Formulation:
  250 mg
Adult prophylactic dose:
  One tablet weekly

Doxycycline
Formulation:
  100 mg
Adult prophylactic dose:
  One tablet daily

Maloprim
Formulation:
  pyrimethamine 12·5 mg, dapsone 100 mg
Adult prophylactic dose:
  One tablet weekly

- Avoid mosquito bites, especially after sunset, when the anopheline mosquitoes that transmit malaria are most active. Long trousers, sleeves, and dresses, netting on windows, and mosquito nets (which may be impregnated with insecticide) over beds all help to prevent mosquito bites.

- Insect repellents may be used on exposed skin and insecticides inside buildings or on breeding sites.

- Mosquitoes should not be encouraged to breed by leaving stagnant water—for example, in blocked drains or around plant pots.

- Prophylactic tablets are often necessary because the above measures, although valuable, are unlikely to be fully effective.

- Take one or two doses of tablets before departure to confirm tolerance and build up serum concentrations of long acting drugs.

- Take the tablets absolutely regularly. The dosages of drugs used for prophylaxis are not normally curative once the infection is established.

- Continue prophylaxis for at least four weeks after leaving an endemic area; all forms of the parasite develop first in the liver and only later re-enter the blood, where most prophylactic drugs take effect.

- Seek medical advice for fever, especially if associated with rigors up to 6 weeks after return or after discontinuing prophylaxis.

Choosing the best prophylaxis

Doses of prophylactic antimalarials for children

Age	Weight (kg)	Fraction of adult dose		
		Chloroquine/ Proguanil	Maloprim	Mefloquine
0–5 weeks		1/8	Not recommended	Not recommended
6 weeks–11 months		1/4	Not recommended	Not recommended
1–5 years	10–19	1/2	1/4 (2–5 years)*	1/4 (2–5 years)*
6–11 years	20–39	3/4	1/2	1/2 (6–8 years) 3/4 (9–11 years)
12 years and over	>40	Adult dose	Adult dose	Adult dose

When both are available, weight is a better guide than age for children over 6 months.
* For children <2 years in areas of chloroquine resistance use chloroquine + proguanil.

Deciding the most appropriate regimen for a particular traveller is not straightforward. There is no perfect antimalarial drug or combination of drugs, only a reasoned choice after the region, the parasites, and the traveller's personal details have been considered. In chloroquine "sensitive" areas, chloroquine is preferred but there are few such areas now, mainly in north Africa, the Middle East, and central America.

In areas with widespread resistant falciparum malaria, it is preferable to take chloroquine *and* proguanil *or* mefloquine on its own. An alternative regimen, chloroquine plus Maloprim (also called Delta–prim), is widely used in parts of southern Africa and Papua New Guinea. Doxycycline is a useful drug where mefloquine resistance is present or side effects preclude its use. All these regimens have their own problems with side effects and breakthroughs.

When there is resistance to prophylaxis

Partial resistance is common

Atypical illness can occur

In "breakthroughs" parasites may be very scanty

Repeated blood films may be necessary

Recrudescence can occur after stopping prophylaxis

Resistance problems—There is increasing resistance worldwide to both the chloroquine plus proguanil and the chloroquine plus Maloprim combinations. Mefloquine resistance is much more unusual but is now present in the Far East, for example, in border regions of Thailand with Myanmar and Cambodia. It has been recognised in Africa, particularly western Kenya and Tanzania.

Despite being less effective in many parts of the world, the chloroquine plus proguanil combination remains popular when other drugs are contraindicated, for example during pregnancy or in infants, or when the traveller is concerned about side effects. Some may also prefer this less effective option for short, up to 2 week, package holidays when illness is likely to occur after return home, when prompt effective treatment should be available. If less effective alternatives are used the risks must be clearly explained. Sometimes it may be appropriate to advise cancelling or postponing a trip, for example if a pregnant woman is planning to backpack in rural Africa.

Suitable choices of anti-malarials are available from specialist centres listed in the final chapter of this book or from the Malaria Reference Laboratory (0171 636 7921).

Areas of low risk—A traveller to areas where there is only a "low risk" of malaria (see table) need take no drug prophylaxis. As with breakthroughs while on prophylaxis, however, the need for early treatment must be emphasised and it may be appropriate to carry empirical treatment to take if medical help is not available. For emergency "standby" treatment, quinine plus doxycycline, mefloquine (if not used for prophylaxis) or Fansidar are suitable. When "standby" treatment has been used, medical advice must still be sought as soon as possible.

Some low risk areas often visited from Britain

- Egypt, Morocco, Turkey, Mexico
- Singapore, Hong Kong, Peninsular Malaysia
- Mainland Philippines, major cities and Bali in Indonesia
- Kathmandu and mountain trekking routes in Nepal
- Bangkok, Chiang Mai, and beach resorts in Thailand
- China, excluding south-west border region and rural parts of the central belt

Side effects of prophylactic drugs—Chloroquine and proguanil can cause nausea which may be eased by taking tablets after a meal. Prolonged use of chloroquine can result in corneal and retinal changes, and the drug should be changed when about 100 g has been taken, which takes about six years at normal adult doses. More common is blurred vision due to visual accommodation problems, reversible when chloroquine is discontinued. Proguanil is an antifolate drug but rarely gives haemopoietic problems in the doses listed. It has been associated with mouth ulcers.

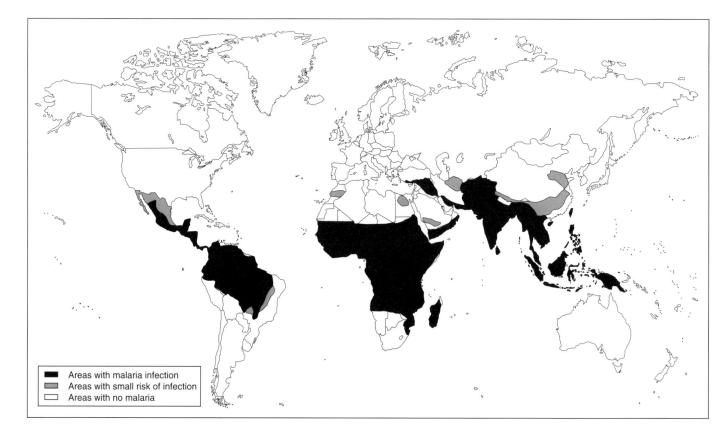

- ■ Areas with malaria infection
- ▨ Areas with small risk of infection
- ☐ Areas with no malaria

Notes on anti-malarial prophylactics

- Chloroquine: resistance common, occasional temporary blurred vision, rarely retinal damage. Use alternative after 5 years. Available as a syrup
- Proguanil: resistance common, very safe, may cause mouth ulcers
- Maloprim: maximum dose 1 tablet weekly. Occasional agranulocytosis
- Mefloquine: avoid in first trimester of pregnancy, can cause neuro-psychiatric side effects
- Doxycycline: avoid in pregnancy and children

Mefloquine can also cause nausea, and sometimes dizziness or psychiatric symptoms. Sulphonamide sensitivity is a contraindication to Maloprim which contains a sulphone (dapsone). Agranulocytosis has been reported with Maloprim when taken in a higher dose, or more often than one tablet a week. Doxycycline can cause photosensitivity.

Both chloroquine and mefloquine are contraindicated when there is a history of convulsions. Proguanil, on its own in areas of low resistance, or else doxycycline, are suitable alternatives.

Emergency "standby" treatment regimens for malaria (adult doses)

- Quinine: 600 mg, 3 times daily for 3 days *plus* doxycycline 100 mg daily for 7 days (Reduce dose if side effects of quinine occur, which are more likely if mefloquine has been used for prophylaxis)
- Fansidar: 3 tablets in a single dose (Resistance is quite common)
- Mefloquine: 500 mg × 2 doses 12 hours apart (Not in pregnancy or if used for prophylaxis: side effects common)

Pregnancy and infancy—The risks from malaria during pregnancy outweigh those from prophylaxis and the usual drugs used are chloroquine and proguanil which have a long reputation for safety. This combination is also considered safe in infants and should be given from birth in high risk areas. Mefloquine is now considered safe in the second two trimesters. Quinine is considered the safest drug for treatment in pregnancy if prophylaxis fails.

Maloprim contains dapsone, which binds to blood protein and is best avoided in neonates when doses can result in higher blood concentrations than expected.

In myasthenia gravis, crises can be precipitated by all the usual prophylactics and treatments. Avoiding exposure may be the only solution. In renal and liver failure, advice from specialist centres should be sought.

Declining immunity

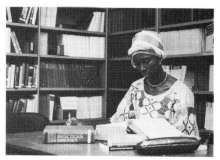

Students visiting Britain may lose their immunity.

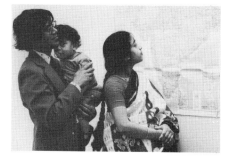

After about 15 years of continuous exposure immunity can develop to the point that infection no longer gives rise to symptoms despite parasites still being detectable in the blood.

Prevention is particularly important in those without, or with declining, immunity which for practical purposes includes those who have never lived in malarious areas and those who have not recently been exposed. This includes, for example, students from Africa who have been in Britain for as little as a year. Pregnancy also makes illness more likely. Having grown up in malarious areas and survived to develop immunity they may not want to start a habit of regular prophylaxis on visits home if they eventually intend to return permanently. Nevertheless, their immunity will be waning and prompt treatment of attacks will be necessary. This may require them to carry a course of treatment if visiting remote areas.

Those who have immigrated to Britain also require special advice. When they left their country of origin, as well as incorrectly believing they had lifelong immunity to malaria, they may have been in a malaria-free area to which the disease has now spread. At present this is a problem for those paying return visits to the Indian subcontinent. Frequently they may be reluctant to take prophylaxis because the relatives they will be staying with do not. The dangers of this must be emphasised.

Failed prophylaxis

Patients, particularly those who have been in malarious areas for many years, sometimes complain of contracting malaria despite prophylaxis. Consequently they may lose confidence in prophylaxis and stop taking precautions, with possibly fatal results.

There are various reasons for "failure".

Prophylaxis against *P falciparum* is less effective against *P vivax* and *P ovale* because these parasites may persist in the liver and produce illness after prophylaxis has been stopped.

If falciparum malaria occurs while travellers are taking prophylaxis it must be established whether they have been taking tablets regularly and in the correct dose. Sometimes a gastrointestinal upset may have resulted in tablets being vomited back or not absorbed properly. Some people confuse prophylaxis with treatment and do not realise that prophylactic doses are not normally curative if the disease has become established. If there is no doubt about compliance or the accuracy of the diagnosis drug resistance must be considered and adjustments made in the recommended tablets.

Finally, the best prophylaxis is not always effective and malaria should be considered whenever fever occurs in someone who has been exposed. Even after apparently successful treatment or prophylaxis, partially resistant falciparum infections may recrudesce during the six weeks immediately after medication has been completed.

> **Prophylaxis sometimes fails. If it does consider:**
> - Poor compliance
> - Drug resistance
> - Poor absorption due to vomiting or severe diarrhoea
> - The illness may not have been malaria
> - Vivax malaria can occur up to 18 months after prophylaxis has been stopped

For further information on malaria prevention see Malaria prophylaxis: guidelines for travellers from Britain. *BMJ* 1995; **310**: 709–14.

The map showing areas of malaria risk is reproduced with permission from *International travel and health. Vaccination and health advice 1996*. Geneva: World Health Organization, 1996.

DURING TRAVEL AND ACCLIMATISATION

Motion sickness

Motion sickness can occur, in order of frequency, during sea, air, road or train transportation. It can also result from rapid movements on cinema screens and in rollercoasters, and is caused by conflict between the body's different motion receptors—visual, vestibular and body proprioceptors. A similar response can occur due to "fear of heights". It is rare in those under 2 years of age.

The symptoms are abdominal discomfort, nausea, malaise, pallor, and sweating, usually followed by vomiting. Lethargy can follow. When the cause persists, as on a ship, adaptation usually occurs after 2 or 3 days.

In those prone to motion sickness the anticholinergic drug hyoscine (Kwells) is a more effective prophylactic than the anticholinergic action of antihistamines, although hyoscine is associated with more side effects, particularly dry mouth, drowsiness, and blurred vision. Because of this it is best reserved for short trips, when a single prophylactic dose will suffice. It is contraindicated in those suffering from glaucoma. Hyoscine skin patches are useful but sometimes difficult to obtain. There is little difference in effect among the many preparations of antihistamines, although their side effects and duration of action vary. Cyclizine is a short acting variety with less sedating effect and can readily be repeated. Promethazine is longer acting, has a low incidence of side effects, and is given as a single daily dose. Alcohol potentiates the sedating effect of all these drugs, and all impair driving ability. Although these oral preparations may still be of some use after symptoms are established, absorption will be haphazard in the presence of vomiting.

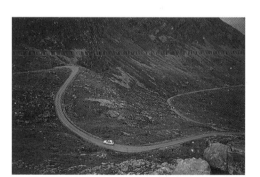

Hairpin bends—a potent cause of motion sickness

Some anti-emetics available "over the counter"

	Adult dose	Effective after (hr)	Duration of action (hr)
Cyclizine (Valoid)	50 mg	1–2	4–6
Hyoscine (Scopolamine)	0·3–0·6 mg	0·5–1	4–6
Promethazine (Avomine)	25 mg	1–2	24–30
Meclizine (Sealegs)	25 mg	2	6–12
Cinnarizine (Stugeron)	30 mg	2–5	6–8

Elasticated wrist bands (Sea Bands) are also available. These contain a firm protuberance that presses against a relevant Chinese acupuncture point. They have no side effects, do not need to be remembered beforehand, and apparently work well in children.

Comfort during travelling is increased for all by choosing the most stable part of the vehicle—between the wings of an aeroplane, in the middle of a boat, or in the front seat of a car; by limiting food and alcohol intake; by adequate fresh air; and by lying down when practicable.

Susceptibility to motion sickness tends to decrease with continued or repeated travel.

Air pressure problems in aircraft

Modern passenger aircraft are not pressurised to the equivalent of atmospheric pressure at sea level because fuselages would have to be much stronger (and hence heavier and more costly) to withstand the pressure difference when flying at a normal cruising altitude of 30 000 feet. A compromise is reached when the cabin pressure approximates to atmospheric pressure at an altitude of 5000–7000 feet. This has two effects: reduction of partial pressure of atmospheric oxygen, and expansion of gases within enclosed cavities.

Reduced partial pressure—Pressure within the fuselage is maintained at about 80 kPa (600 mm Hg), resulting in an alveolar PO_2 of 10 kPa (75 mm Hg). This reduces the haemoglobin oxygen saturation by only about 4%, so has little effect on the average person. Those with severe respiratory or cardiovascular disease, severe anaemia, or sickle cell disease, or recent episodes of myocardial ischaemia and cerebral infarction are, however, at risk and should travel only if it is essential. Smoking (active or passive) during the flight will reduce haemoglobin oxygen saturation even further. Pregnant women over 35 weeks' gestation are usually not allowed on long flights because of the possibility of the onset of labour, and there is a risk of fetal hypoxia. Puffy feet are common, due both to the reduced pressure and the continual sitting. Shoes are best removed, the feet exercised, and occasional walks up the aisle are recommended.

Expansion of gases—The volume of enclosed gases will increase by about one third. In its most innocent form this may lead just to "popping" of the ears and abdominal distension, but it may put at risk recent gastrointestinal surgical wounds. Carbonated drinks will exacerbate this. Clearly those with blocked sinuses or middle ears will suffer, and recent middle ear operations may be stressed especially during descent. Similar problems can occur in transit through underground tunnels, as in the recently opened Channel Tunnel between England and France. Any unabsorbed pneumothoraces will expand.

> ## Contraindications to air flights
>
> Severe anaemia
> Severe otitis media and sinusitis
> Acute contagious or communicable disease
> Recent myocardial infarction
> Uncontrolled cardiac failure
> Recent cerebral infarction
> Peptic ulceration with haemorrhage within 3 weeks
> Simple abdominal operation within 10 days
> Major chest surgery within 14 days
> Contagious or repulsive skin diseases
> Wired fractures of mandible
> Mental illness without escort and sedation
> Pregnancies after 35th week (long journeys) or 36th week (short journeys)
> Introduction of air into body cavities within 7 days
> Neonates (within first 2 days)
> Terminal illness
> Gross behavioural disturbances (e.g. serious drunkenness)

Fear of flying

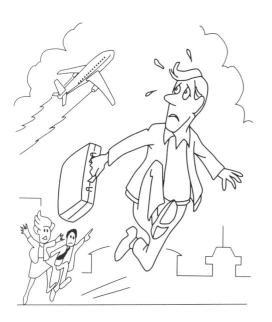

This is a very real difficulty for some travellers and in an international business world can have job implications. An estimated 9 million people in Britain suffer anxiety through to severe panic attacks. Milder degrees of fear may be helped by good preparations, informing the cabin staff in advance and perhaps taking a mild tranquilliser. Heavy smokers may find non-smoking flights difficult.

When there is a serious problem a psychological approach such as cognitive behaviour therapy may be necessary.

The atmosphere in aircraft cabins

As well as problems related to cabin pressure described above, cabins have to be kept dry and this can lead to dehydration, often aggravated by heavy alcohol or caffeine intake. The skin becomes dry and often flaky. Dry air can lead to nasal congestion. The combination of a dry cabin and a smoky atmosphere can be very unpleasant, even for regular

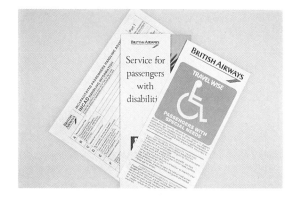

smokers. There are times when smoking is forbidden, such as during take off and landing, and although there is no convincing evidence that serious disease has resulted from smoke in cabins, increasingly airlines are banning smoking altogether on short and sometimes long haul flights.

Fitness to travel—Specific advice about the fitness to travel of individual patients and the facilities available can be obtained from the medical departments of the airlines concerned. A standard form is used by most airlines with parts to be filled in by the ticket agent and the attending physician. Wheelchairs are the most commonly used facility but stretchers and supplementary oxygen are also available.

Acute contagious and communicable disease, as listed in the contraindications to air travel, is not strictly defined but is not meant, in practice, to include mild upper respiratory infections like the common cold. Cases brought to the attention of the airlines' medical departments are decided on their individual merits. There have been recorded outbreaks of both influenza and tuberculosis originating in aircraft cabins.

Jetlag

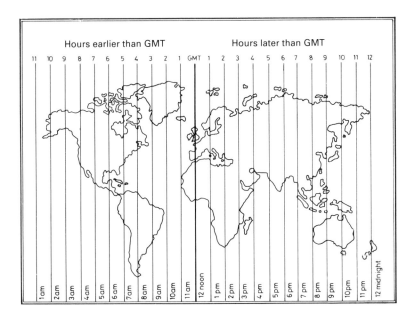

Air travel enables passengers to cross time zones more rapidly than the body's innate circadian rhythms take to adjust. Many rhythms exist but those most upset relate to sleep and wakefulness, hunger, and defecation. It has been estimated that crossing five time zones (five hours' time difference) is necessary for jetlag to be appreciable. Adjustment takes longer (up to 50% longer) if the flight is eastwards rather than westwards—that is, when the day of travel is shortened rather than lengthened. Adjustment may take longer with increasing age and is exacerbated by lack of sleep during the actual travelling, the stress of travelling, and alcohol.

Most travellers are not prepared to undertake fastidious diets, or adjust artificially their day and night cycle, or both, before travel in order to shorten jetlag.

The practical implications of this are to recognise that performance after arrival will be substandard and sleep patterns disturbed, with full adjustment taking up to a week. Once this is recognised allowances should be made. Sleep on the plane is recommended, aided if necessary by a mild sedative; no heavy commitments should be booked for the first 24 hours, especially if a sharp intellect is required; alcohol intake should be limited; and sleep should be of normal duration.

The metabolism of drugs within the body varies through the day but a change in time zones will probably be of consequence only to diabetic subjects. They should be recommended to keep on home time for medication and meals, when practicable, until they can adjust on arrival at their new destination (see page 50).

Acclimatisation after travelling is related not only to time zone differences but also to adjusting to changes in climate, geographical features such as altitude, and culture.

Preventing jetlag

- Rest before departure
- On the flight get maximum sleep
- Stretch and exercise as much as possible to aid circulation and prevent swollen ankles
- Drink plenty of water or soft drinks to counteract the dry cabin atmosphere
- Alchohol and caffeine increase dehydration
- Jetlag is made worse by a hangover!
- Breaking very long journeys halfway with a stopover can be helpful
- Have as few commitments as possible on the first day after arrival

Cruises

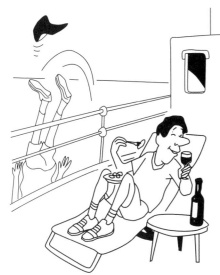

Sea sickness can be helped by rest, limiting alcohol intake, and anti-sickness tablets. The centre of a ship is less prone to rolling movements.

Unaccustomed overindulgence with food and alcohol is common. Maximum use should be made of exercise facilities.

Food and water facilities during shore visits may be poor, making some vaccinations advisable. There may be a risk of malaria when on shore, in port or even from mosquitoes that have "come on board ship". In most Asian, Mediterranean, South and Central American ports short daytime visits ashore should not pose a serious risk, but it is wise to check that emergency treatment is available on board ship before deciding not to take preventative tablets. Entering ports in sub-Saharan Africa (except for South Africa) usually warrants taking prophylaxis.

A yellow fever certificate may be required if visits ashore are planned. Check for each country concerned.

Sun, heat and cold

Sun and heat are one of the most common problems affecting travellers, who may be going on holiday specifically to enjoy the sun. Exposure to ultraviolet radiation can cause sunburn and heat stroke. Both are more common at altitude and at sea or when rays are also reflected by snow.

> **Exposure to sun increases the risk of skin cancer, especially in fair skinned people**

Exposure to sun can lead to premature ageing of the skin and an increased risk of melanoma and other skin cancers. There is a greater risk among those who are fair skinned, or on certain medications such as tetracyclines and diuretics. Babies and children are always at high risk.

Fifteen minutes in the midday sun is usually sufficient initial exposure to Mediterranean sun for the average British traveller. Adjustment can be made by gradually increasing the period of exposure, avoiding the midday sun (usually between 11 am and 3 pm), wearing a wide brimmed hat and sunglasses and using an appropriate sun protection cream (higher factors giving greater protection). Manufacturer's instructions need to be followed carefully and the cream may need to be reapplied frequently.

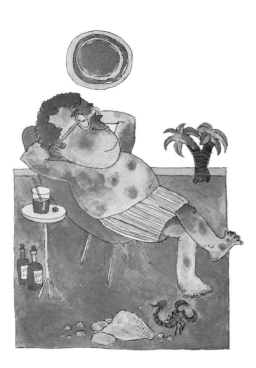

Increased sweating is inevitable in warmer climates and initially this is inefficient, leading to excessive loss of water and salt. Unless severe exertion is undertaken, the loss of salt is adequately countered by the addition of extra table salt to meals. Increased fluid intake, often several litres a day, is necessary but should not be solely of tea, coffee, or alcohol. The colour of urine is a rough and ready guide and should be kept pale. Considerable adjustment of sweating mechanisms, leading to lower sweat volume and lower sweat sodium concentration, occurs within five days and is complete within two weeks. Normal salt intake can then be resumed. The elderly, very young, obese, and those with extensive skin disorders take longer to adjust. Light, loose clothes, particularly cotton ones, encourage the evaporation of sweat and hence more efficient cooling.

Exposure to extreme cold is likely to be anticipated, as when mountaineering, and suitable clothing is essential. Hypothermia can kill within a few hours and the onset is often insidious, with lethargy, shivering, falling, blurred vision, vague behaviour and ultimately confusion and coma. Children and young adults are especially vulnerable.

Cold injury can damage the skin and its extreme form is frostbite, with loss of digits. Sunburn from excessive ultraviolet radiation can aggravate cold injury on exposed skin.

Altitude

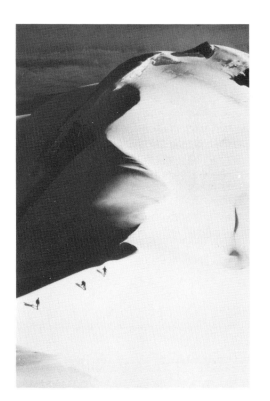

Acute mountain sickness affects most people who live at low altitude and ascend to 2400 metres and above. About 5% are severely affected. The severity is related to the altitude reached, speed of ascent, and concurrent exertion. Susceptibility varies greatly from person to person and those who do suffer may well develop similar symptoms on future trips to high altitudes. In its mild form the common symptoms are headache, weakness, anorexia, nausea, vomiting, and vertigo. With increasing severity these symptoms merge into those indicative of cerebral or pulmonary oedema—namely severe constant headache, retinal haemorrhages, gross lassitude, confusion, inappropriate shortness of breath, cough, and cyanosis.

A slow ascent (above 4000 metres this should be as little as 150–300 metres per day, and 400 metres per day from 2400 to 4000 metres) is the best prophylactic measure to modify symptoms. This can be aided by sustained release acetazolamide 500 mg nightly. The acetazolamide is thought to counter the respiratory alkalosis induced by hypoxia and thus allow increased ventilation. Peripheral paraesthesia is a common side effect. Nifedipine 20 mg three times daily also seems to have a prophylactic effect.

Should mild symptoms develop, rest at that altitude is recommended. The onset of the severe symptoms mentioned above is often insidious but rapid recognition and prompt descent are essential to avoid unnecessary rescues and deaths. Dexamethasone, oxygen, and nifedipine may be of help in allowing prompt descent to be made safely.

It must be noted that acclimatisation to high altitude is lost within 1–2 weeks, after which symptoms will recur with a new ascent.

Some airports, especially in South America, are already at high altitude and may cause difficulties, especially for those with pre-existing cardiorespiratory problems. Specialist advice prior to travel should be sought.

PERSONAL MEASURES FOR PREVENTING ILLNESS WHILE ABROAD

With immunisations completed, and with antimalarial and possibly antidiarrhoeal tablets in hand, the departing traveller may be tempted to think that no further health precautions are necessary. Few of these preliminary measures are fully effective, however, and unexpected diseases may occur. Many illnesses could be prevented by simple precautions—in particular with water, food, sexual habits, and personal hygiene. Care over sunbathing and unfamiliar surroundings that lead to accidents have been mentioned already.

Drinking water

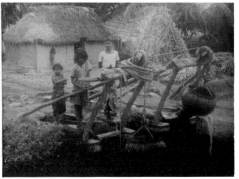

Drinking water from unprotected wells is risky.

At present three-fifths of the world's population are estimated to have inadequate supplies of drinking water. Contamination of drinking water with living organisms is a major cause of illness amongst travellers. In Britain we drink water straight from the tap and rarely consider that water may be a source of disease. Most short stay tourists are unlikely to face a shortage, but when this occurs the water may carry a higher proportion of impurities and pathogenic organisms because of concentration.

Water pollution is usually caused by human and animal excrement. The likelihood of this must be considered. For example, is the tap water supply from surface sources? This is more likely to be contaminated than that from artesian or protected deep wells. Does the water supply pass through an efficient purification plant? There may be no easy way of discovering this, particularly for short term travellers. Most package tours are arranged to hotels where the tap water is reliable or filtered boiled water is provided for drinking and cleaning teeth, but special care should still be taken when drinking out.

Escherichia coli gastroenteritis, giardiasis, cryptosporidiosis, shigellosis, amoebic dysentery, hepatitis A, typhoid, and cholera may all be water borne. When the cleanliness of a water supply is in doubt, the best means of sterilising drinking water is by boiling or good filtration. Iodine (five drops/l) or tablets, left for 20 minutes—longer in cold climates, and chlorination with tablets (follow manufacturers' instructions), are helpful alternatives although second best because of difficulties in controlling these methods by the occasional user. Some cysts and hepatitis A virus can be resistant especially to chlorine. Reliable filters are increasingly available and are becoming less expensive. They may be appropriate for long term expatriates or those on prolonged overland journeys or safaris.

Cysts can remain viable on utensils washed in contaminated water, later infecting food and drinks taken from them. Water used for brushing gums and teeth, washing foods, and making ice may also be a source of infection. Bottled water and other drinks are usually safe, especially if carbonated, but locally produced drinks, including some in bottles, may not have been sterilised. Babies who are breast fed are unlikely to be infected until water is drunk and weaning begins, and the value of breast feeding should be emphasised. If bottle feeding is used scrupulous attention must be paid to hygiene both with water for mixing feeds and with utensils.

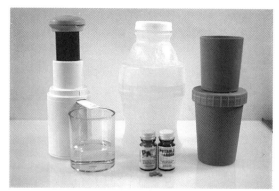

Boiling or filtering with a reliable filter are the best ways of purifying water for personal use.

Swimming and water associated diseases

Avoiding infections that enter the body by penetrating the skin

Schistosomiasis, hookworms, and **strongyloides** spread through fresh water or moist ground contaminated with human or animal urine or faeces. A specific snail host is necessary for spread of schistosomiasis.

- Avoid skin contact with fresh water in endemic areas—for example, ponds, lakes, and rivers. Swim only in protected swimming pools and safe sea water
- Avoid drinking infected water
- Wear protective footwear when walking in soil, particularly if it is damp or waterlogged.

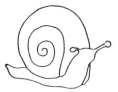

The main hazard from swimming is accidents—diving into shallow water or slipping on wet surrounds to swimming pools. If the water in swimming pools smells of chlorine the risk of contracting ingested infections is probably slight, but hepatitis A and cyst borne infections are still possible. The Mediterranean Sea has gained a reputation for pollution because much sewage and industrial waste empties directly into the sea, which has only a minimal tide flow, limiting its dispersal. The direct risk to bathers is, however, small and usually limited to the immediate surrounds of the waste outlets, where solid matter is present.

The traveller to the tropics must be aware of the dangers of water associated diseases such as schistosomiasis, which is prevalent where defective sanitation combines with the presence of fresh water weed and the snail vector. Tour operators and hosts may play down the risk of swimming at the local beauty spot. Local advice should be sought before swimming at sea as there may be sea snakes, which are especially prevalent in coastal waters around Asia and in the western Pacific, and other sea creatures such as jelly fish, some of which can cause irritating rashes or occasionally fatal stings. More accidents are due, however, to lack of respect for sea currents and use of floating air beds as well as the inexperienced using canoes and small boats.

Food and alcohol

Points to remember

- Unless you are sure of the purity of the local water supply don't drink it without boiling it first or using iodine tablets or a reliable iodine based filter. This also applies to water used for ice cubes and for cleaning teeth
- Bottled water is usually safe, as are hot tea and coffee, beer, and wine
- Unpasteurised milk should be boiled before use. Local cheeses and ice cream are often made from unpasteurised milk, and care should be taken with both. Buy ice cream from larger firms only
- All meat should be cooked thoroughly and eaten hot whenever possible. Avoid leftovers
- Be wary of shellfish
- Eat only cooked vegetables and avoid salads
- Peel all fruit, including tomatoes
- Wash hands thoroughly with soap and clean water before eating or handling food, and always after using the toilet.

When in doubt, miss it out!

Most food-related illness is due to either infection or a change in the amount or type of food, which may upset those, for example, with oesophageal reflux or gall bladder problems. Infection may originate in the food—for example, tapeworms or toxoplasmosis—or be introduced by dirty hands or through washing foods with impure water. Some foods are particularly prone to contamination, and care should be taken, as indeed it should be in Britain.

Poultry is a common source of salmonella and campylobacter infections, especially when eaten cold. All meat of uncertain origin should be thoroughly cooked and eaten hot whenever possible. Some fish contain toxins in their flesh. This is more common in fish from tropical seas and sometimes occurs only at certain times of year. Gastrointestinal and neurotoxic symptoms may occur. In addition to being responsible for similar toxin-mediated effects, shellfish, particularly bivalves (cockles and mussels), concentrate micro-organisms through their food filtering mechanisms and are renowned for transmitting hepatitis A. The traveller will have to depend on local advice but is wise to avoid seafoods when in doubt. Vegetables and fruit may have been manured with excreta or handled with dirty hands, but cooked vegetables are usually safe, and fruit can be peeled. Salad vegetables are harder to clean and are a frequent vehicle for infection.

Many people drink more alcohol than usual while on holiday, and in hot climates this may aggravate heat exhaustion as well as resulting in a laissez-faire attitude towards risks from food, drinks, and sexually transmitted diseases.

Unpasteurised milk may convey tuberculosis, brucellosis, Q fever, salmonellosis, and campylobacter infection, and boiling is essential if there is doubt about sterility. This applies to goat as well as cow or buffalo milk, and milk or cream used in preparing yoghurts and cheeses.

Personal hygiene

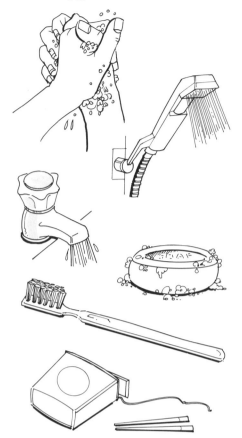

Sanitation and water supply go hand in hand. Water closets are obviously inappropriate where there is not enough water for drinking and washing. The inexperienced traveller may find dry and "crouch" type toilets difficult to use, and washing rather than using toilet paper is standard in many countries. Thorough hand washing before eating as well as after going to the toilet is firmly recommended.

A shower is generally a more effective way of cleaning the body than a bath, but showers and air conditioning systems may be responsible for spreading *Legionella pneumophila*, the organism responsible for Legionnaire's disease. It is most likely to cause infection when disseminated in an aerosol, possibly in association with free living amoebae, and inhaled. It is difficult to give the traveller specific advice on how to prevent infection, but there is evidence that hotels and similar institutions are becoming more aware of the problem. Adequate chlorination of all public water supplies and increasing the temperature of hot water supplies should reduce the incidence of this infection, and running a shower for a short while before using it may help to flush out organisms that tend to accumulate around taps and shower heads. In Britain it was first recognised in tourists returning to Scotland from a package tour to Spain, and a third of the cases occurring in Britain each year are imported.

Human tuberculosis and leprosy are widespread in tropical areas and are thought to be transmitted principally through sputum and nasal discharge, respectively. Those repeatedly exposed, as in a hospital, are at greatest risk from these infections. Safe disposal of infected material should be encouraged.

Care of the teeth and gums should not be neglected after having made sure before departure that they are in good condition. Dental sticks and floss are valuable, especially when there is doubt about the sterility of tooth brushes and water.

Sexually transmitted and blood borne infections

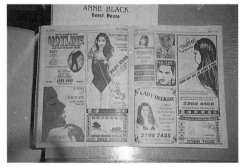

Sexual contact through the "yellow pages".

- Beware of casual sex
- Use a condom
- Alcohol encourages sexual risk taking

Contents of a typical kit for prevention of blood borne infection

Assorted syringes and needles
Materials for cleansing skin
Waterproof dressings and plasters
Needles for suture of the skin
Steristrips
(Intravenous cannula)
(Blood/intravenous fluid giving set)
(Plasma expanders)
Certificate for customs purposes

If the traveller indulges in casual sex the risk of infection with a sexually transmitted disease, which may be caused by a resistant organism, is high in many parts of the world. Gonorrhoea and syphilis may cause serious long term disability, particularly if effective treatment is delayed. Hepatitis B and HIV are also spread sexually.

It is clear that HIV infection is now widespread and although prevalence is high among homosexual groups and intravenous drug users in "Western countries", it is, on a global scale, primarily spread by heterosexual contact. High proportions of the general population in many parts of Africa are infected, and AIDS is common. Infection is also widespread in other countries, including Asia and South America, and illnesses resulting from immunocompromise are now appearing on a wide scale. High proportions of sex workers are infected in these areas. The message must be that casual sexual intercourse is risky worldwide, and condoms provide good but not complete protection.

Contracting HIV infection from blood and blood products is largely preventable by screening these for infection before use, but although such tests are widely available their cost restricts their use in some countries. In addition, antibody tests alone will not detect infected blood during the "window period" one to three months after infection has occurred.

Blood transfusions and immunoglobulin products should be used only when they are essential, and it can be helpful if travellers know to which blood group they belong in advance, and ideally also their HIV status. Travellers can make up their own, or buy commercially prepared, travel packs that contain disposable needles and syringes for use in an emergency, rather than depend on local—possibly unsterile—equipment. An advantage of a bought set is that it is usually supplied with a certificate listing its contents and the reason for its purchase, which is useful for customs clearance.

Bites, stings and skin care

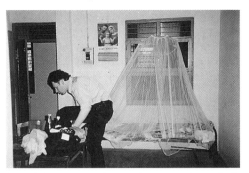

Remember to practise putting up your net before departure.

Remember to take a mosquito net

- Portable nets are often difficult to obtain abroad
- Those with one suspension point are easiest to erect
- Choose one impregnated with insecticide
- Re-impregnate nets every 6 months after washing

Insect repellents

- Those containing di-ethyltoluamide (DEET) are most popular
- Different strengths are available for adults, children, and clothing
- Minimise their use by covering up with loose, airy clothing
- Follow the instructions about re-applying
- Eucalyptus and neem oil based repellents are also effective

---

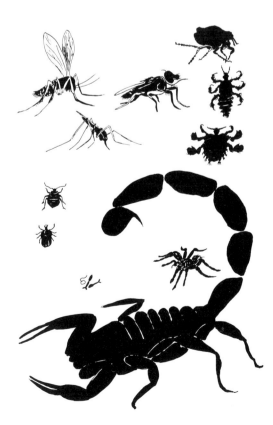

Mosquitoes, sandflies, tsetse flies, and other biting insects cause much inconvenience because of local reactions to, and secondary infection of, the bites themselves as well as from the infections they transmit, such as malaria, leishmaniasis, and trypanosomiasis. Local reactions usually become less of a problem as time passes because some immunity develops. Some people, however, develop hypersensitivity. Mosquitoes bite at any time of day, but most bites occur in the evening. A common mistake is to travel to hot countries equipped only with short sleeves and nothing to cover the legs with in the evenings. The chat in the cool of the evening may then be spoilt by the constant biting.

Various insect repellents are available, and ones containing diethyltoluamide are most widely used. They have to be applied to all exposed areas and last for only a few hours: impregnated elastic bands (Buzz Bands) can be slipped over ankles or wrists, and are effective over a longer period. Most people constantly exposed find that appropriate clothing, window netting, and mosquito nets over beds are more practical. Small *eye flies* are difficult to control and may transmit agents causing conjunctivitis.

Cool footwear such as open sandals with no socks or tights reduces the chance of tinea pedis but exposes the feet more to mosquito bites and injury, with the risks of secondary infection and, in the unimmunised, of tetanus. Feet in contact with water or damp soil may be penetrated by pathogenic *leptospires*, *hookworm larvae*, and the *cercariae* of schistosomes.

Other unexpected sources of skin reactions, usually limited to erythema or urticaria, include *caterpillars*, *blister beetles*, *mites*, *bed bugs*, and *sea creatures* such as jellyfish. Campers and those walking in the country may be bitten by ticks, which should be removed promptly and completely. They can be avoided by keeping to paths. They transmit infections such as tick typhus, encephalitis, and borreliosis (Lyme disease). *Leeches* can be troublesome and potentially dangerous if they attach themselves internally or are so numerous as to cause anaemia. For those likely to be exposed to these creatures protective clothing is valuable and chemical impregnation can be considered.

Although infestations such as *scabies* and *head lice* are seen in Britain, they may cause problems for travellers, particularly those living rough or travelling overland in varied accommodation with limited washing facilities. Such travellers often come from social backgrounds where these parasites are unfamiliar.

The size of a *spider* bears no relation to its danger, and *scorpions*, most of which are nocturnal, make walking with bare feet after dark risky. Shoes should be examined before they are put on in case something is resting inside. *Snakes* often shelter under vegetation, among rocks, or sometimes in termite nests. They normally bite humans as a defensive reaction to being disturbed. Poisonous snakes include the elapids (landsnakes with short fixed fangs), seasnakes, and vipers, which probably cause the most deaths. If snake bites are going to produce symptoms they usually do so within 12–24 hours. The various *lizards* which abound in warm climates are generally harmless. In some domestic settings they help keep down mosquitoes and flies.

Dogs and cats abroad should not be petted unless they are known to be healthy. We are fortunate in Britain in not having indigenous rabies but this is not the case in Europe, the Americas, and most tropical areas, the most notorious of which are Asia and tropical Africa. Children particularly may have a strong urge to pet stray animals, and this must be prevented.

Bites and skin injuries should always be cleaned and dressed with special care until healing takes place. They easily become infected in tropical climates.

First aid for bites and stings is covered in the next chapter.

Some health risks for which there are no currently available effective vaccines

Cholera, bacterial dysentery and "food" poisoning
Of world-wide distribution, these illnesses are normally contracted through contaminated drinking water and food. The responsible organisms in water usually are destroyed by chlorine, iodine or boiling. Thorough cooking will destroy them in food. Hand washing before eating is important.

Giardiasis and amoebic dysentery
These causes of diarrhoea are contracted through contaminated food and water. They are spread by cysts which resist drying and can survive for a long time, for example, on contaminated dishes and cutlery. The cysts are resistant to chlorine but iodine or boiling usually destroys them in water and thorough cooking in food.

Dengue (breakbone fever)
Widespread especially in Asia, Central and South America, and the Middle East, dengue causes a feverish illness with headache and muscle pains like a bad, prolonged, attack of influenza. There may be a rash. A severe haemorrhagic form can develop, especially in children. Dengue is spread by mosquito bites.

Schistosomiasis (bilharzia)
Widespread in Africa, schistosomiasis causes infection of the bowel and bladder, often with bleeding. It is caused by a fluke whose life cycle requires fresh water snails. It is contracted through the skin from fresh water contaminated with urine or faeces. Paddling or swimming in suspect fresh water lakes or slow running rivers should be avoided.

Onchocerciasis (river blindness)
This infection occurs in West and Central Africa and can cause a skin rash with intense itching due to microfilaria usually months or sometimes years after exposure. Occasionally the eye can be affected. It is spread by the bite of a small black fly found close to fast running water where it breeds. Camping near rivers should be avoided and precautions taken against bites.

Bancrofti filariasis
Widespread in Asia, Africa, and South America this is the infection that can cause gross lymphoedema of the legs, arms or genitalia. Deformities only occur after repeated infections. It is caused by microfilaria and spread by mosquito bites against which precautions should be taken. It is not usually a problem for the short-term traveller staying in good accommodation.

Tick borne typhus
This infection is most common in southern Africa and is spread by tick bites. It causes a feverish illness, usually mild, often with a rash. The bite is usually obvious. There is a risk if walking through long grass or scrubland. Ticks can be brought home by domestic animals.

Leishmaniasis
This infection, usually contracted in the Middle East and Asia, is spread by the bite of an infected sandfly. It can cause a slowly growing skin lump or ulcer and sometimes a serious life-threatening fever with anaemia and weight loss. Infected dogs are carriers of the infection. It is not usually a problem for the short-term traveller staying in good accommodation.

Social and psychological adaptation

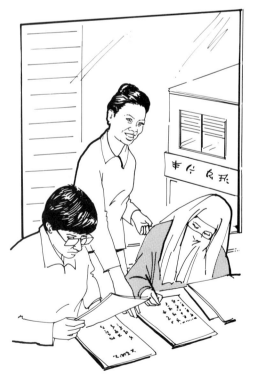

Awareness that living overseas will demand changes in lifestyle does not necessarily make adaptation easier. The numbers of people who return for psychiatric reasons and who cut short contracts working abroad indicate that many have difficulty in adapting. Similar problems may contribute to the high alcohol consumption and common complaint of headaches among holidaymakers. Separation from relatives and friends with whom problems are normally shared, language and currency differences, and adjusting to the image that local people may have of the expatriate may all cause difficulties. Bargaining, using public transport, and accepting domestic help may be stressful. In professional relationships the role expected of the foreigner may vary from that of a respected counsellor to that of an intruder.

The package tourist may be able to get help from a representative of the tour company and also knows that even if things become difficult he or she will soon be returning home. Those spending longer abroad may find it helpful to seek specific advice before departure about the area to be visited, although personal experiences and requirements are unlikely to be identical. For example, some people like to take with them familiar possessions, while others prefer to buy items abroad, where they may be cheaper and more appropriate. Some organisations, such as Voluntary Service Overseas and missionary societies, arrange courses before departure or periods of adaptation while overseas in the company of experienced expatriates. If an adviser or friend can greet the newcomer on arrival he or she may help to overcome many seemingly difficult domestic problems early. A conscious and determined effort to learn the local language is valuable, and a musical, dramatic, or other social skill which can entertain others is likely to be appreciated where entertainment is not dominated by mass media. Many parents find their children lead them quickly to new friendships.

Finding out where medical help is available before it is needed can prevent unnecessary anxiety, especially for those who have a disability or have children travelling with them.

Often problems can be anticipated by a thorough social and psychological assessment before final travel plans are made.

FIRST AID WHILE ABROAD

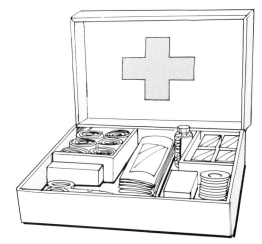

The traveller is exposed to organisms not prevalent at home, has to adjust to different climates and cultures, and experiences trauma of the accidental, biting, and stinging varieties. Most illnesses are mild and will not require medical consultation, but some will be severe and may require attention after return home.

Travellers often do not know how to seek medical advice while abroad and may be reluctant to do this because of language difficulties, cost, doubts about the quality of service, or remoteness. English speaking doctors are, however, available in most cities and hotel receptions, tour company couriers, British embassies, and consulates will know where to obtain medical advice. With the widespread prevalence of HIV infection, consideration also has to be given to the sterility of available medical equipment and the safety of blood transfusion, for instance, after a traffic accident.

Although an illness may be minor or self limiting, it can still cause distressing symptoms amenable to simple treatment. For this reason most travellers carry some drugs and first aid equipment. The content of any first aid box will vary both with the worries and the intent of the traveller. We will consider only basic essentials and not discuss the specialist requirements of groups such as those making expeditions to remote areas. We have assumed that severe or persistent symptoms lead to self referral to a doctor.

Traveller's diarrhoea, respiratory tract infections and fever

Gastrointestinal illnesses

Diarrhoea affects many people travelling from areas with high standards of public hygiene to areas with lower ones. The incidence of travellers' diarrhoea among British travellers is higher in those going to Africa or the Indian subcontinent, for example, than in those going to Mediterranean countries. The causes have been described elsewhere.

Prophylaxis—Some broad spectrum antibiotics are effective in reducing the incidence of traveller's diarrhoea. Antibiotics are not routinely recommended because of their potential for selecting antibiotic resistant bacteria, and because of side effects such as rashes or mental confusion with ciprofloxacin. Antibiotics benefit those who need to be fit for a short period, such as businessmen, entertainers, and athletes, and should be considered for the elderly, and those who are immunocompromised or have disabilities such as inflammatory bowel disease. Bismuth subsalicylate is thought to reduce the intestinal secretion induced by toxins and hence is effective prophylaxis and symptomatic treatment. It has become available in Britain (Pepto-bismol) but is bulky to carry in the dose recommended—60 ml four times daily.

Treatment—Patients whose diarrhoea is associated with any of the following symptoms should seek prompt medical advice: prostration, persistent vomiting, high fever, the passage of blood and mucus from the rectum, and frequent copious watery stools in the young child. Vomiting associated with the onset of diarrhoea in milder illness usually does not persist. It is essential to replace fluid loss, particularly in the young and elderly. Over a short period even water is satisfactory

---

Travellers' diarrhoea

- Drugs sometimes used for prophylaxis
  A 4 aminoquinolone such as ciprofloxacin
  Bismuth subsalicylate
  Doxycycline

- Drugs for treatment
Antidiarrhoeals	Antimicrobials
Loperamide	Ciprofloxacin
Lomotil	Trimethoprim

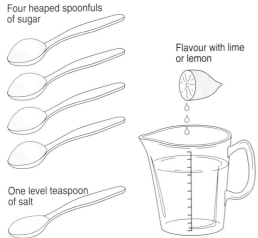

Four heaped spoonfuls of sugar

Flavour with lime or lemon

One level teaspoon of salt

One litre of water

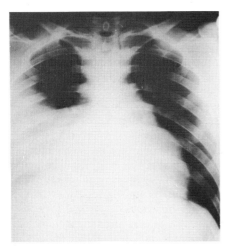

Severe respiratory symptoms may be due to Legionnaires' disease.

though a solution containing electrolytes, such as fruit juice, weak soups, or diluted milk, is preferable. A homemade electrolyte preparation can be made from one level teaspoonful of salt and four heaped teaspoonfuls of sugar, dissolved in 1 litre of sterile or boiled water. This should not taste salty and may be flavoured.

Reduction of stool frequency and abdominal discomfort can be achieved in adult patients by Lomotil (diphenoxylate with atropine) but this drug should not be given to infants or used frequently in children. Loperamide (Imodium) reduces intestinal secretion induced by toxin as well as bowel motility, without any central nervous system depression (as with Lomotil). A syrup is available for children over 4 years of age. These drugs can increase nausea and vomiting. Trimethoprim, and ciprofloxacin have been shown to reduce symptoms when given early.

Traveller's diarrhoea lasts on average three to four days. Chronic symptoms require further evaluation. Immunity to enterotoxinogenic *Escherichia coli* is thought to last about six months, but as traveller's diarrhoea may be caused by many organisms further episodes are to be expected when staying in high risk areas.

Respiratory illnesses

Respiratory infections are common worldwide (including tropical areas), particularly in the cooler months. As at home, they are usually viral in origin, and mainly affect the upper respiratory tract. They should not be routinely treated with antibiotics. Ephedrine nasal drops help prevent disturbed sleep, particularly in the younger child. Symptoms warranting further advice are high fever, prostration, confusion, rapid respiratory rate, or localised chest pain when pneumonia or Legionnaires' disease are possibilities. If a cough persists tuberculosis should be excluded.

Febrile illnesses

Symptomatic treatment with paracetamol or aspirin is appropriate unless fever is accompanied by severe symptoms or persists for more than two to three days. Rigors should always prompt medical advice, and emergency self treatment of malaria is discussed in the chapter on malaria prevention.

Although there are many serious causes of fever requiring accurate diagnosis and appropriate treatment, brief febrile episodes with mild systemic complaints of headache, anorexia, and malaise occur commonly within the tropics. Most are presumed to be of viral origin.

Risks from unsterile needles

- Avoid use of unsterile needles and infusion sets
- Consider taking a sterile equipment pack
- Remain within range of good facilities if blood may be needed (e.g. if pregnant, have an ulcer or a bleeding tendency)
- Make sure insurance covers repatriation in emergencies

HIV, hepatitis B and C infections may be spread by unsterile needles, used for injections, infusions, manicure, tattoos, or acupuncture. Blood transfusion is a risk, especially in areas of high prevalence. Major centres in all countries usually have sterile equipment and blood donations are tested for such infections, though local knowledge of their whereabouts may have to be obtained rapidly—from the local British embassy or consulate, for example. In more remote areas travellers must ensure that if equipment is not from sterile packages it is properly sterilised by boiling or chemical disinfectants. In such areas blood transfusion should only be accepted when absolutely necessary and when "plasma expanders" will not buy sufficient time for the traveller to be moved or tested blood obtained. This predicament emphasises the need to have adequate medical insurance that will ensure rapid repatriation if necessary.

Commercial packs of needles, syringes, and infusion sets are available for travellers, but as mentioned above, this equipment is readily sterilised anyhow. Bigger packs containing plasma expanders are also available but have a limited role except perhaps for expeditions where medical or nursing help is on hand.

Risks from excessive sun and heat

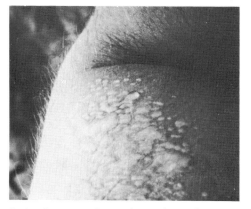

Sudamina: sweating under sunburn about to peel.

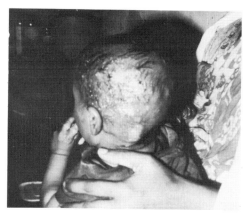

Prickly heat.

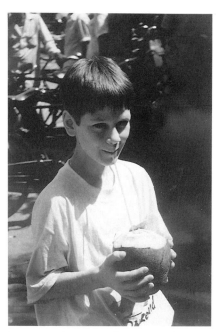

Coconut milk is a useful source of sterile rehydrating fluid.

Sunburn—The local skin damage caused by overexposure to the sun's radiation will vary from shortlived erythema and tenderness to oedema and blistering accompanied by pronounced systemic upset. Further exposure should be avoided until symptoms have settled, remembering that radiation can penetrate thin clothes, clouds, water and even shade, by reflection off bright surfaces such as snow and water. Cool showers and "after-sun" lotions provide local relief. Bursting of blisters encourages secondary infection.

Prickly heat (*miliaria rubra*)—This intensely irritating rash occurs after sweat ducts have been blocked by keratin plugs. Subsequent sweating leads to small vesicles being formed in the sweat ducts which, with further sweat output, rupture into the epidermis, inducing a local inflammatory response. The rash appears as areas of erythema within which are small papules. The initial duct blockage occurs in flexures or where clothes fit closely to the skin, as around the waist. In infants it also occurs on the scalp. Both indigenous and expatriate children are commonly affected in hot, moist climates and secondary staphylococcal sepsis is common.

Treatment is aimed at preventing sweating by reducing exertion, taking cool showers, dusting with talc and wearing light, loose cotton clothing. Calamine lotion and oral antihistamines help relieve the pruritus. Excessive use of soap is thought to encourage further attacks. Severe attacks may warrant transfer to a cooler climate.

Heat exhaustion results from heavy sweating and inadequate or inappropriate fluid replacement. It is often a problem for those performing unaccustomed exercise during acclimatisation. There are body deficits of salt and water and the symptoms vary according to which predominates. Both have a slow onset, with increasing malaise, headache, light headedness, and tiredness. Those mainly water deficient complain of thirst if heat exhaustion is mild, but increasing severity leads to clouding of consciousness. Sweating still occurs and there may be slight fever. Signs of dehydration and hypotension may be present. Rehydration (by mouth if the patient is conscious) and cooling lead to rapid recovery. Those mainly salt deficient feel less thirst and remain rational, though suffering more intense lethargy, vomiting, and muscle cramps. Oral rehydration should initially be with salted fluids; one level teaspoonful of salt to 500 ml water is adequate but moderately salty soup or Bovril is more palatable. Salt in fresh lime juice is remarkably refreshing and widely drunk in south east Asia. Fresh coconut milk is sterile and contains minerals and potassium. Further attacks of heat exhaustion can be prevented by less exertion during acclimatisation, adequate fluids, and added salt in meals. Travellers should take plentiful fluids on their journeys. Muscle cramps due to salt deficiency can occur on their own.

Heatstroke—Should the sweating mechanism fail to cool because the sweat glands are fatigued or damaged, as in those with chronic prickly heat, extensive skin disorders, or severe water deficiency, then a rise in body temperature is inevitable, leading eventually to heatstroke. The word "stroke" implies the suddenness of the collapse although there may have been a short period of irrational and perhaps hyperactive behaviour before. The body temperature is above 40 °C, the skin dry, and the patient usually unconscious. Cooling is urgently required, preferably by spraying with cold water and fanning. Excessive cooling is prevented by stopping these measures when the temperature falls to 39 °C. Other causes of fever and unconsciousness have to be considered.

Skin trauma, bites, and stings

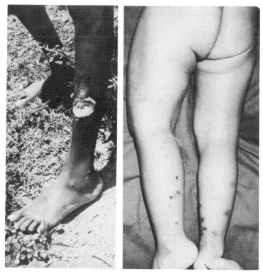

Chronic ulceration (left) should be specifically diagnosed. Right: papular ulticaria from bites.

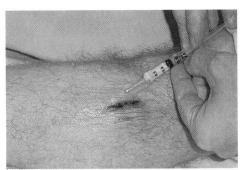

A traveller with a dog bite receiving immunoglobulin to the surrounding tissue.

Snake bites

- Wipe off excess venom
- Reassure strongly, give alcohol or sedative and adequate analgesia
- If bite is on limb apply broad bandage, preferably crepe, firmly to whole limb. Do not occlude arterial supply. Do not release
- Keep patient still while removing him to hospital
- Take snake if already killed, but do not chase
- Observe patient closely for 12 hours

Animal bites and licks

- Wash lesions copiously and thoroughly with soap and water. Apply 40% alcohol (most spirits) or stronger, or iodine. Do not suture immediately
- If owner of domestic animal available, ask whether animal vaccinated and ask to see last vaccination certificate. Exchange addresses and telephone numbers for contacting should animal become unwell in next two weeks
- Seek local medical advice regarding vaccination
- Inform local police
- Inform own doctor on return

Minor trauma to the skin can be a considerable hazard, especially where hot, moist climates encourage secondary infection and delay healing. All such wounds should be promptly cleaned, treated with an antiseptic ointment and covered with a dry, aerated dressing or adhesive plaster. Infected wounds may need an antibiotic if there is evidence of spreading infection such as a widening area of erythema, enlargement of draining lymph nodes, or systemic complaints. Pus should be allowed to drain freely. *Staphylococcus aureus* and *Streptococcus pyogenes* are the common secondary infecting agents. Chronic ulceration should be specifically diagnosed.

The physical nature of trauma from bites and stings is complicated by the effects of various inoculated poisons leading to local inflammatory or cytotoxic reaction, perhaps with systemic features if severe.

Mosquito and other insect bites commonly cause a pruritic papule when these insects are first encountered. Lesions in women are often more severe with central vesiculation and a wide surrounding zone of erythema. Gradual desensitisation occurs over the first few weeks as further bites occur. Some symptomatic relief may be obtained from oral antihistamines and local calamine ointment if lesions are severe. Although antihistamines can be allergenic when applied topically many find them effective when rubbed immediately on the bite.

Bee and wasp stings may also be eased by local use of an antihistamine or by an icepack once any remnant of the sting of the bee has been removed.

Ticks should be removed completely with a firm pull vertical to the skin surface while gripping them as close to the skin as possible, ideally with tweezers so as to avoid leaving behind the mouth parts.

Leeches can be pulled off or removed by putting salt, alcohol, or strong vinegar around their mouths, or by heating their bodies with a burning cigarette.

Spiders and scorpions—Most bites or stings cause only local irritation but occasionally intense local pain occurs. Analgesics and icepacks give symptomatic relief. Rarely systemic symptoms occur, particularly in younger patients, and further advice should be sought. In some areas some antivenoms are available.

Snakes—Many bites by venomous snakes cause little or no envenoming but bites by all snake varieties cause severe fright. Systemic absorption of toxin is usually along the lymphatics and this is slowed by compression with a firmly applied bandage. After viper bites severe envenoming is characterised by pronounced spread of local swelling within one to two hours, accompanied by shock and a haemorrhagic tendency. In elapid bites, such as cobras, the other main venomous group, severe illness can be expected if shock and neurological signs develop within one hour of the bite. Specific antivenom is usually reserved for those developing systemic or severe local symptoms.

Sea creatures—If spines are present they should be removed, and relief from the often severe local pain can be achieved by soaking in water as hot as is bearable. Any undischarged nematocysts of jelly fish are neutralised with vinegar or removed with dry sand.

Cats, dogs, and wild animals—In an area endemic for rabies all bites or licks should be considered suspect. Immediate cleansing of the wound is important and should be thorough. If pre-exposure vaccination has not been received, post-exposure vaccination should be commenced immediately, ideally accompanied by antirabies immunoglobulin to the wound site and parenterally. If pre-exposure vaccination is up to date, a booster dose should still be given but this can be arranged with less urgency (within 5 days). (See also chapter on immunisation.)

First aid box

Items that may be considered for a first aid/medicine box

- Paracetamol or other analgesic/antipyretic
- Loperamide for diarrhoea
- Dressings, adhesive plasters and steristrips
- Promethazine as an anti-emetic and mild sedative
- Sunscreen and "after sun" lotion
- Fucidin ointment for infected sores
- Antihistamine cream for itchy bites
- A nasal decongestant may be useful prior to flying

Also advisable in some circumstances
- Anti-malarials* (except chloroquine and proguanil)
- Antibiotics* (e.g. augmentin, ciprofloxacin and metronidazole)
- Standby emergency treatment for malaria*

Other items useful for prevention of illness
- Iodine tincture/tablets for water sterilisation
- Insect repellents
- Water filter
- Mosquito net
- Kit for prevention of blood borne infection
- Condoms
- Prophylaxis for mountain sickness*

(* medical prescription only)

Many will have their own opinions on what medications they wish to carry. Considerations vary with likely risks. Possible choices for a trip during which at least some time is spent in remote areas is shown opposite. *Promethazine* is antiemetic and can be used to prevent travel sickness. Its antihistamine action can ease irritation or urticarial lesions resulting from bites and it is also useful as a mild sedative. The self administration of *antibiotics* without medical advice is not routinely recommended but it is not difficult to envisage situations where advice is not available for some days. We would take ciprofloxacin, clavulanate-amoxycillin (Augmentin) or doxycycline. They would be expected to improve most cases of bacterial tonsillitis, acute otitis media, lower respiratory infections, urinary tract infections, and skin sepsis, with ciprofloxacin being used primarily for traveller's diarrhoea. Metronidazole may also be useful, and if appropriate an emergency course of anti-malaria treatment. *Oil of cloves* is useful for pain of dental origin when rubbed locally over the area of tenderness. The following guidelines on self treatment may be found helpful.

Some guidelines for the adult traveller on emergency "self-medication"

Professional advice should be sought when you are ill but sometimes this is impossible if you are in remote places. Most of the medications described below are only available on prescription but your doctor may be prepared to give you courses to take away with you. You should make sure you understand clearly, through discussion with your doctor, when to use each medicine, the correct dose and what side effects might occur.

- **Sudden onset, but not severe, diarrhoea**
  Avoid dehydration by drinking plenty of clear fluids (water, juice, coconut milk)
  Loperamide may help if diarrhoea continues or if you have colic. Taking too many may make you feel sick and constipated later on.

- **Sudden onset, more severe, diarrhoea and/or feeling unwell**
  Avoid dehydration by drinking as above. You can also use *dioralyte* rehydrating solution. If you have fever, profuse diarrhoea, or blood in the motion take a short course of *ciprofloxacin*. (Augmentin and doxycycline may also help.) Use *loperamide* as above.

- **Persistent diarrhoea (may be due to giardiasis or amoebic infection)**
  Diarrhoea sometimes grumbles on, often with nausea, anorexia, a lot of wind and frothy smelly motions. Medical attention should be actively sought, but if delayed you could try *metronidazole* (*Flagyl*).

- **Malaria**
  There are many causes of fever but malaria can be very serious and need prompt treatment. Remember malaria occurs occasionally even if you are taking your anti-malarial tablets correctly.
  You may get severe shivering followed by sweating. A clue is that between fevers you may not feel too bad. If in doubt consider fever to be due to malaria until proved otherwise.
  You must try to get a doctor's help, but if this is delayed take *quinine* 600 mg (2 tablets) three times a day for 3 days *and doxycycline* one capsule (100 mg) daily for 7 days at the same time. (*Quinine* can give buzzing in the ears, especially if you have been taking *mefloquine* for prevention—if this happens reduce to two doses of 600 mg per day.)
  Fansidar on its own (3 tablets only, all at once) is an alternative treatment but occasionally fails to cure—quinine rarely fails.

- **A bad sore throat, cough with green spit, badly infected skin sores or bites**
  Take *augmentin* (*doxycycline* is an alternative).

- **Itchy bites**
  Antihistamine cream may help. Remember *antihistamine cream* itself sometimes causes a rash. *Promethazine* is an oral antihistamine (anti-allergy drug and mild sedative). It may help if lots of bites stop you sleeping.

- **Infected bites and skin sores**
  Use *fucidin ointment* (or iodine) on the sores.

INFECTIONS ON RETURN

What infections are imported?

With the speed of modern travel, infections contracted abroad may only be in their incubation phase at the time the traveller returns home, and a history of recent travel when dealing with unexplained illness is as important as details about a patient's occupation or current medication. Sometimes a period of many years is relevant.

The numbers of cases of imported infection as confirmed by laboratories only partly reflects the problem since they tend to emphasise bacterial diseases such as salmonellosis and other food poisonings. It is important to realise that totals of confirmed "imported" infections do not take into account infections occurring while travellers are abroad. These are very difficult to document accurately. We do not know, for example, how many long term expatriates die while abroad from malaria or contract diseases with short incubation periods such as cholera or dengue.

Malaria is very important because the malignant form, due to *P. falciparum*, can be rapidly fatal. The total number of cases imported into Britain has stayed steady recently at around 2000 per year but the proportion of falciparum (malignant) malaria has markedly increased in line with increased travel to sub-Saharan Africa.

Giardiasis is a common cause of grumbling alimentary symptoms that is often not immediately recognised.

Enteric fever continues to present, usually contracted in the Indian sub-continent, and often in immigrants revisiting their home country, inadequately immunised. Increasingly serology is allowing specific diagnosis of protozoal and helminthic infections: for example, schistosomiasis, filariasis, dengue, and typhus. Special problems recently have been the increasing number of people contracting schistosomiasis in Malawi and travellers to the Far East contracting dengue.

Of concern is the increasing number of HIV infections contracted abroad, usually heterosexually.

Infections such as cholera, rabies, plague, and Ebola or Lassa fever, despite receiving a lot of publicity, are very unusual.

Groups affected reflect the seasonal pattern of travel, with most imported infections occurring during the British summer and autumn months. Most travellers are between 15 and 60 years of age and the more experienced, including regular business travellers staying in good accommodation, tend to get fewer problems.

Some imported diseases have an importance out of proportion to their incidence, such as falciparum malaria, Legionnaires' disease, the haemorrhagic fevers. Early suspicion of the diagnosis is essential in these diseases to establish optimal treatment. Other infections, such as typhoid fever, have public health implications when excretors handle food.

Some of these conditions are within the everyday experience of general practitioners in Britain. Others are unusual and this may lead to failure or delay in making the diagnosis. Referral to an infectious or tropical disease unit is often advisable both for speed and ease of unusual investigations and to supervise treatment which may need drugs not commonly used in Britain.

Fever

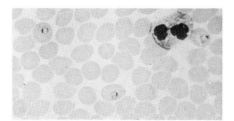

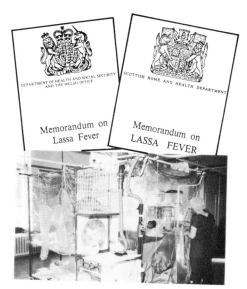

Remember to ask for blood film examinaton.

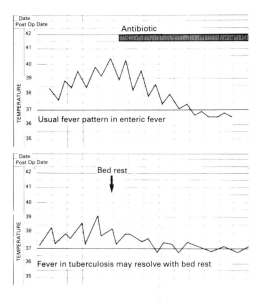

Memorandum on
Lassa Fever

Memorandum on
LASSA FEVER

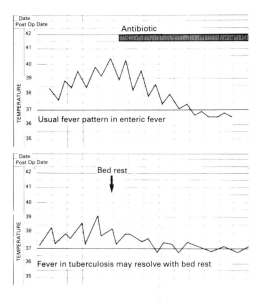

Usual fever pattern in enteric fever

Fever in tuberculosis may resolve with bed rest

Could fever be due to falciparum malaria?

Any patient with fever who has been exposed could have falciparum malaria. Associated symptoms of diarrhoea, jaundice, or confusion must not distract the physician from this possibility. Prompt treatment is necessary to prevent the cerebral, renal, and haematological complications which can rapidly cause death in the non-immune. Consultation with a specialist and admission to hospital for assessment are usually indicated. In recently contracted falciparum infection the fever tends to be irregular and unpredictable, in contrast to an established vivax infection, where fever usually occurs on alternate days.

A blood film examination must be arranged immediately. It is important for the examination to be done by someone with experience of the disease.

Chloroquine remains reliable treatment for vivax but not for falciparum infection because of drug resistance. In an ill patient with falciparum malaria it is safer to use quinine usually combined with doxycycline or Fansidar. If there is delay in getting laboratory confirmation, then treatment must be commenced empirically.

Could fever be due to viral haemorrhagic fever?

The rare possibility of viral haemorrhagic fever should be considered in all patients with fever who have been in Africa south of the Sahara during the three weeks before the onset of their symptoms. Lassa and Ebola fever can both have a high mortality. Primary contacts of a human case are at risk when exposed to blood, body secretions, and urine. Lassa is predominantly a disease of west Africa and Ebola of central African countries. It is important to seek advice from a specialist in infectious or tropical diseases before embarking on investigations or allowing a possible case to come into contact with others. When haemorrhagic fever is definitely suspected the patient is managed along nationally accepted guidelines using secure laboratory and isolation facilities. In England and Wales the local Consultant in Communicable Disease Control and in Scotland and Northern Ireland the local consultant in Public Health Medicine should be notified immediately. This procedure is to prevent unnecessary contact with other people that would occur if a patient was referred to hospital in the usual way. In practice, suspected cases are rarely confirmed and many of these patients have illnesses such as malaria.

Some other causes of fever

Typhoid fever usually presents as a septicaemic illness, and fever has often been present for several days before the symptoms prompt investigations. This illness illustrates the importance of performing a blood culture in unexplained fevers as it is positive in 90% of untreated cases. *S. typhi* from Asia is now often multidrug resistant.

In conditions such as *tuberculosis* or *brucellosis*, where the onset of illness may be more insidious and the course prolonged, patients may be unaware of their fever. A rise in temperature in the evening or night is followed by sweating, which may be the predominant complaint. Fevers of this type can settle transiently with bed rest alone, which may confuse the unwary. Dengue is an acute severe flu-like illness which is common in Asia, central and south America. "Breakbone fever" describes associated muscle pains. A rash and haemorrhage can occur.

Influenza and other common causes of fever are also contracted by travellers. Too casual a clinical diagnosis of such illnesses, however, may delay recognition of less familiar but more serious infections.

Bacterial (usually toxin mediated) intestinal infections

> **Some causes of diarrhoea in the returned traveller**
>
> **Usually mild**
> E. coli (entero-toxinogenic)
> Unaccustomed spices and oils in diet
>
> **May be severe**
> Shigella dysentery
> Amoebiasis
> Salmonellosis
> Cryptosporidiosis
> Campylobacter infection
> E. coli 0157 (verotoxinogenic)
> Yersinia and Aeromonas infection
>
> **Often grumbling or chronic**
> Giardiasis
> Amoebic colitis
> Cyclospora infection

"Traveller's diarrhoea" due to *Escherichia coli* will usually have begun while abroad and is self limiting. If symptoms persist after return other causes should be considered.

Salmonella, Shigella, Campylobacter and *Yersinia* infections may all be associated with prolonged symptoms and blood in the stools.

Profuse watery diarrhoea within a few days of returning from abroad may be due to *cholera*. Adequate replacement of fluid and electrolytes is life saving, and there is evidence that a short course of aminoquinalones can shorten severe and more toxic illnesses. Drug resistance is common to more "traditional" antibiotics.

Protozoal infections

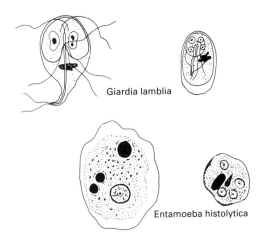

Giardia lamblia

Entamoeba histolytica

Giardiasis commonly causes prolonged symptoms. Often one or two loose stools are passed each morning, accompanied by unpleasant flatus. Abdominal discomfort and nausea may persist throughout the day and be exaggerated by alcohol. Anorexia is common and travel sickness may be easily provoked. The infection is diagnosed by finding cysts or trophozoites in the stools. If stool examination is negative protozoa may be found in jejunal juice or on small bowel biopsy, but unless there is malabsorption or another reason for these investigations empirical treatment with metronidazole or tinidazole is usually tried first.

Amoebic dysentery may have an acute or subacute onset and immediate examination of freshly passed stools is necessary to reveal motile amoebae. Ulceration and stricture formation give persistent symptoms. In chronic disease stool examination and other investigations will be necessary to make the diagnosis and exclude malignancy. Amoebic antibodies are helpful in diagnosing *amoebic liver disease*. A liver which is tender to percussion should suggest this diagnosis. Steroids are dangerous in untreated amoebic infection.

Cyclospora infection has recently been recognised as a cause of chronic diarrhoea, especially in the Indian sub-continent and Nepal. It may respond to co-trimoxazole.

Other causes of diarrhoea

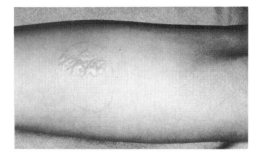

Strongly positive Mantoux reaction.

Symptoms of malabsorption, particularly in travellers from Asia, should suggest *postinfective tropical malabsorption* (tropical sprue).

Abdominal pain and fever are features of *tuberculosis* affecting the bowel or abdominal lymph nodes. There is often a delay before the diagnosis is considered. Barium and chest radiography may show no abnormalities, but the Mantoux reaction is usually strongly positive. Stool cultures may be positive. A trial of antituberculous treatment after other non-invasive investigations have been completed can help to prevent an unnecessary exploratory laparotomy.

When alimentary symptoms are present but an infective cause is not found the following questions should be asked.

(1) Has there been exacerbation of previously existing disease, such as diverticulitis, irritable bowel syndrome, peptic ulceration, or ulcerative colitis?
(2) Is the primary cause outside the bowel? Malaria may cause diarrhoea and vomiting. Infections elsewhere may provoke gastrointestinal hurry, particularly in young children.
(3) Are the symptoms the result of medication? Some antidiarrhoeal agents aggravate nausea and vomiting, and antibiotics may change bowel flora, causing diarrhoea or candidiasis.
(4) Is there disaccharidase deficiency or protein intolerance? This is most likely in young children but may affect all age groups. It is usually self limiting but may require a temporary change in diet.

Intestinal *roundworms* may produce abdominal discomfort but are often just noticed in stools or vomit. *Strongyloides stercoralis* may cause pain, abdominal distension, and diarrhoea in the early stages of the infection. *Hookworms* and *Trichuris trichuria* infection may cause anaemia if infection is heavy. Pruritus ani from *threadworms* is common. The dangerous tapeworm is the pork tapeworm, which can cause cysticercosis.

A high eosinophilia suggests invasive helminthic disease such as strongyloidiasis, or schistosomiasis. When *schistosomiasis* affects the bowel the stool is usually formed but is sometimes blood stained. Snips of rectal mucosa may show the characteristic ova. When the urinary tract is affected blood and ova may be present in the urine. Serological examination is helpful particularly in asymptomatic infection. All these infections should be treated even though light parasitisation rarely causes serious complications.

Filarial infections also cause eosinophilia, the most common being due to Bancroftian filariasis that usually presents with fever. Onchocerciasis presents with pruritis and skin rashes or nodules. Loa-loa can cause typical "Calabar swellings".

Most of these infections can be symptomless or present years after exposure.

No organisms found
- Giardia is a small bowel infection—cysts may be scanty
- Medication or pseudomembranous colitis
- "Post-infective" irritable bowel
- Inflammatory bowel disease
- Malabsorption or tropical sprue
- If there is fever—could it be malaria?

Helminth infections

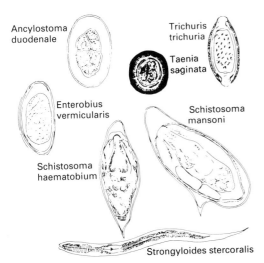

Jaundice

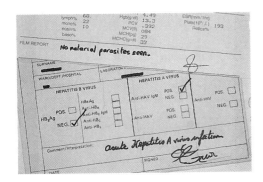

The two commonest infective causes of jaundice in the returning traveller are viral hepatitis and malaria. Haemolysis due to *falciparum malaria* must be excluded first because of the need for urgent treatment. Both hepatitis A and B are normally afebrile illnesses once jaundice has appeared and can therefore be distinguished clinically from malaria.

The severity of an *acute* hepatitis A or B infection is related to age, with children usually getting milder illnesses. Despite the high carriage rates of hepatitis B surface antigen in some tropical countries, hepatitis B usually affects only those who use intravenous drugs, are exposed sexually, get tattooed, are occupationally exposed or receive blood or blood products. The diagnosis of hepatitis is confirmed by raised liver enzyme and the infecting agent determined by the presence of hepatitis A, IgM antibodies or hepatitis B serological markers. Recently large outbreaks of hepatitis E spread by the faecal–oral route have occurred in Asia and Africa.

Respiratory symptoms

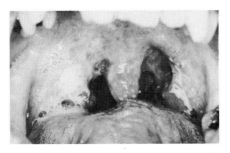

In a returning traveller phanyngitis could be a feature of diphtheria or Lassa fever.

Respiratory symptoms are common in travellers. Exposure to unfamiliar infectious agents, dust, and excessive alcohol consumption may be contributory factors. Most respiratory illnesses are mild, but special attention should be given to throat infections and pneumonias.

Throat infections—A "toxic" patient with an adherent membrane on the palate and fauces may have diphtheria. Culture of a throat swab is important even in milder cases of sore throat when there is a recent history of travel, because if toxigenic *C. diphtheriae* is identified, prophylaxis or immunisation of contacts, or both, has to be considered. A sore throat in a febrile patient recently returned from west Africa warrants specialist help because of the possibility of Lassa fever.

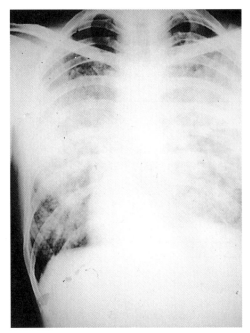

Erythema migrans (Lyme disease).

Pneumonia—Legionnaires' disease usually presents with pneumonia but it is a multisystem disease that often includes gastrointestinal and neurological features. Confusion, hallucinations, dysarthria, and other cerebellar signs are pointers to the diagnosis. Empirical treatment is necessary because the diagnosis is usually only confirmed later by serology. Tuberculosis and particularly pneumocystis pneumonia, presenting with hypoxia, minimal chest signs, and diffuse shadowing on radiography, raise the question of HIV infection if there are no other predisposing factors.

Neurological symptoms

Headaches were second only to diarrhoea in a recent survey of common symptoms experienced by travellers. Stress, heat, alcohol, prophylactic medications as well as fever are possible causes. Mefloquine can cause dizziness. Confusion, hallucinations, and coma are signs of serious disease, and *malaria* or *typhoid fever* may be the cause. Similar symptoms with pneumonia should suggest *Legionnaires' disease*.

Unexplained fever, vague mental changes, and isolated cranial nerve palsies are common presentations of *tuberculous meningitis*. *Trypanosomiasis* may present similarly when it reaches its cerebral stage.

Poliomyelitis and other enteroviral infections must be remembered as causes of aseptic meningitis. Encephalitis due to arboviruses or spirochaetes (Lyme disease) may have been contracted by those exposed to mosquitoes or ticks, respectively.

Rabies may cause unusual neurological symptoms. By this stage treatment is very unlikely to be effective, but modern vaccines can be used successfully if given soon after exposure. A frequent problem "on return" is advising someone who has been bitten abroad, usually by a dog or cat. If someone has been bitten by an animal in an infected area an international telephone call to try to confirm whether the animal remains alive 10 days after the bite can be reassuring. This may also prevent vaccine being used unnecessarily (see also page 38).

Countries reported free of animal rabies in 1996

Australia	Ireland
Bermuda	Japan
Bulgaria	Malta
Caribbean Islands (excluding Cuba, Grenada, Haiti, Puerto Rico, Trinidad)	Mainland Norway
	New Zealand
	Pacific islands
	Papua New Guinea
	Portugal
Gibraltar	Sweden
Iceland	United Kingdom

Skin disorders

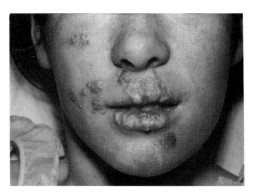

Herpes simplex with secondary impetigo

Herpes simplex may be reactivated by exposure to sunlight.

Chronic skin disorders include persistent sores or septic spots after mosquito bites, fungal infections, and infestation with scabies.

Sometimes a maggot emerges from a sore or abscess after a visit by the tumbu fly. The skin granuloma of cutaneous leishmaniasis is transmitted to man by the bite of an infected sandfly. It can appear within days or be delayed for a year or more.

Cutaneous larva migrans (due to the animal hookworm) is most often seen in visitors to the Caribbean, and erythema migrans due to Lyme disease can follow tick bites, especially in Europe and North America.

In a patient with fever, rashes uncommon in Britain include the maculopapular rash of typhus, the "rose spots" on the trunk in enteric fever, and the lymphangitis of filariasis.

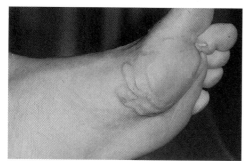

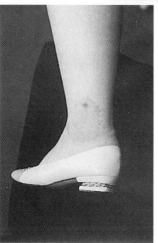

Tuberculosis must be excluded in those with erythema nodosum. Transient urticarial and erythematous rashes occur with filariasis, onchocerciasis, and chronic strongyloidiasis. Pruritis can also be due to skin infestations by lice or scabies, animal hookworm which causes an itch localised track usually on the feet, or as a non-specific feature of HIV infection. Hypopigmentation or anaesthesia may be due to leprosy.

It is wise to arrange a biopsy of any unexplained skin lesion which may have been contracted in tropical areas.

The check-up after returning from abroad

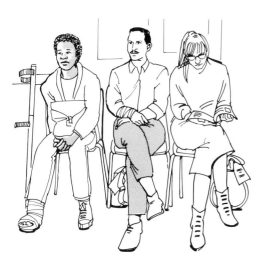

A returning traveller may not feel unwell but may be worried about having contracted an infection that could cause problems later on. This is particularly understandable if the traveller has been to a tropical country, been exposed to poor environmental conditions, insect or animal bites or been at risk of blood borne or sexually transmitted disease. A good history and examination is important which should include details of countries visited, duration of stay, illness occurring while abroad, any residual symptoms such as weight loss, occupational risks, exposure to food and water borne diseases, bites, injections, risky sexual activities, and psychological problems. Weight loss, if there is no underlying illness, often improves rapidly with a healthy diet.

Immediate screening investigations might include a full blood count to check for anaemia and eosinophilia, chest radiography, and a stool examination for ova, cysts, and parasites. An eosinophilia may be due to invasive helminthic or fluke infections such as stronyloides, Bancrofti filariasis, loa-loa or schistosomiasis. If there has been weight loss, radiography may help to exclude tuberculosis and ova of roundworms or other intestinal helminths may be seen on stool microscopy.

Some infections may only declare themselves after months or sometimes years (see chart of "incubation" periods). Blood films for malaria are likely to be negative until there are symptoms. If there has been exposure to schistosomiasis, serology and a urine examination can show evidence of infection in the absence of symptoms. Skin snips and a "provocation test" with di-ethylcarbamazine may be needed after known exposure to onchocerciasis. Usually these tests should only be undertaken after consultation with a specialist who can also help with interpretation of the results and treatment.

If there has been possible exposure to HIV infection, experienced counselling and possibly HIV testing may be appropriate.

"Culture shock" on return is a very real problem, in particular for those who have spent long periods abroad. Finding employment, friends, new schools, adjusting to a more "materialistic" and often impersonal society can be stressful, and depression is not uncommon.

Some firms and organisations organise their own post-travel screening for employees. Individual travellers may seek advice initially from their general practitioners and specialist advice can be sought from infection or tropical disease units.

Some points to consider

- Countries visited
- Environmental conditions experienced
- Illnesses which occurred while abroad
- Exposure to infections that may present "late"
- Occupational risks
- Psychological problems
- HIV counselling

The immigrant or refugee

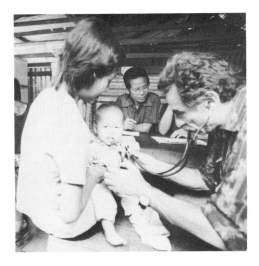

People from countries with limited medical facilities may have seen previously healthy relatives die rapidly with symptoms such as cough or diarrhoea. They may therefore be unduly anxious over what may seem to the doctor to be minor complaints. The help of a sympathetic interpreter is important in evaluating these symptoms and in preventing medicines being taken incorrectly.

Illnesses in their incubation phase as well as established disease may be imported by these groups, as they may be by any traveller from overseas.

Evidence of *pulmonary tuberculosis* can be looked for on a chest radiograph but other forms are not so accessible to screening. Abdominal, bone, urinary, lymph node, and meningeal tuberculous disease may be insidious in onset, difficult to confirm, and require a high index of suspicion.

Bowel parasites may have been accepted as normal.

Hepatitis B surface antigen carriage is common in some parts of the world such as the Far East. There is an increased incidence of cirrhosis and hepatoma in chronic carriers.

Malaria poses special problems for immigrants or temporary visitors. Immunity present on arrival may have declined by the time they return home for a holiday and they may therefore suffer a symptomatic infection.

Fungal infections of the skin such as tinea versicolor are often found.

HIV infection must be considered if there are signs of immunocompromise.

TRAVELLERS WITH EXISTING HEALTH PROBLEMS

When a traveller has an existing health problem a medical consultation before departure can be especially valuable. If the intended lifestyle abroad is likely to aggravate existing illness it may be appropriate to advise that the trip should be cancelled. Usually, however, the advice will be on how to adapt the trip to the patient's abilities, on suitable immunisations and pre-travel arrangements, and on contingency plans for any problems that may arise. The earlier a consultation takes place the easier it will be to be prepared.

The emphasis in this section is on living in tropical areas, where, as well as climatic stresses, drugs, medical facilities, and transport may be in short supply. Problems that may occur in transit in pressurised aircraft and on cruises have been discussed previously.

Emotional and psychiatric disorders

Despite recent changes in overseas living conditions such as more frequent home leave, illnesses with a psychiatric basis still account for many repatriations on medical grounds. There is some evidence that people with personality disorders are more likely to be sent abroad or want to work there, perhaps to escape problems at home. Assessing whether an intended trip is psychologically appropriate is difficult, but an attempt is worthwhile, especially for those intending to live abroad for long periods. It can be helpful to interview spouses and children, on occasions independently. Some firms and organisations make their own psychological assessments of an individual's suitability for an overseas post. Culture shock sometimes has to be experienced to be understood and a short preliminary visit to an intended new work situation may help to identify whether problems are likely.

It may be necessary to seek specialist advice—for example, if the patient has a history of psychotic illness or the intending traveller is currently on psychotropic medication. Remember mefloquine is contraindicated when there is a history of convulsions or psychiatric illness.

Heart disease

The stresses of adapting to new surroundings may increase symptoms of cardiac ischaemia and hypertension. Hot climates may aggravate postural hypotension resulting from the use of antihypertensives, and diuretics may make the salt depletion that occurs during acclimatisation to hot climates more severe. Once this initial period is over, however, living abroad is not usually harmful. Remember proguanil can upset anticoagulation with warfarin and mefloquine aggravates bradycardia in those on β blockers.

Gastrointestinal disorders

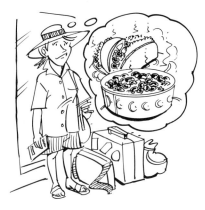

Hernias, haemorrhoids, and pain of dental origin which may have been tolerated at home are usually best treated before departure.

Symptoms from peptic ulceration are less common among expatriates than previously, because of more effective management, but the availability of emergency surgery and blood transfusion must be considered in case complications should occur. Alcohol and spiced foods may also exacerbate symptoms from oesophagitis and oesophageal reflux. Hypochlorhydria, concurrent taking of antacids, and previous gastric surgery predispose to gastrointestinal infections, including typhoid.

Bowel infections can make the management of chronic disorders such as ulcerative colitis and Crohn's disease more difficult. There is evidence that relapses may be provoked by intestinal infective agents. Similarly, patients with the irritable bowel syndrome may expect an increase in symptoms and take longer than others to recover from travellers' diarrhoea and specific infections such as giardiasis and amoebic dysentery.

Respiratory disease

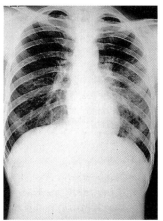

Obstructive airways disease.

Possible problems in pressurised aircraft have already been discussed. Also travel to high altitudes can initially lead to poorer oxygenation and cause difficulties in those with pre-existing lung disease.

There is no escape in the tropics from the many respiratory infections prevalent in temperate countries. In general, they should be no more severe than they would be at home, although secondary bacterial infection may be more common. The response of asthma to changes of climate and surroundings is unpredictable. People with chronic obstructive airways disease tend to find life in the tropics detrimental, perhaps because of dust and increased smoking. Legionnaires' disease is more likely to be life threatening in those with pre-existing lung disease.

Remember to consider both influenza and pneumococcal vaccination and that the influenza season in the southern hemisphere is from May to September.

The immunocompromised

The immunocompromised

Remember to avoid live vaccines, including BCG

Other active vaccines may not produce an optimal response

Malaria may be fulminant after splenectomy

More people are now travelling after organ transplants

Travel related infections may be more severe

There are increasing numbers of people travelling who are immunocompromised due to medication for lymphoproliferative disorders or following renal and cardiac transplants. As with those who have HIV infection, the increased risks of infection must be clearly explained. Extra care must be taken to avoid food-, water-, and insect-borne diseases. Adequate supplies of medication must be taken and the availability of medical facilities at the destination should be determined in advance. The importance of increased doses of steroids during illness and the dangers of dehydration must be made clear. It must be remembered that the response to vaccinations may be poor in the immunocompromised and immunoglobulin, for example, may be preferable to active vaccination against hepatitis A. Live vaccines are usually contraindicated and the importance of malaria prevention must be emphasised.

Sometimes it is necessary to discourage travel when the risks are substantial and medical facilities will be poor. Insurance to cover repatriation is important and there may be increased premiums.

Post splenectomy

The danger of fulminating pneumococcal infection and other bacterial infections after splenectomy is well recognised. It is accepted practice to vaccinate routinely against pneumococcal infection and administer prophylactic antibiotics in circumstances which would include being away from medical facilities while overseas. Meningococcal and haemophilus type B vaccination should also be considered. Malaria is usually fulminant in those with no spleen, so much so that travel to hyper-endemic areas with multi-drug resistance should be firmly discouraged. When exposure is unavoidable, protection against mosquito bites, scrupulous attention to prophylaxis, and "prompt treatment" must be ensured.

Renal failure

Immunocompromise may be present and the advice given above is important. Heat, diarrhoea, and vomiting may precipitate acute onset of chronic disease. Doses of anti-malarials may need to be adjusted and advice from the patient's renal physician before plans are made is prudent even with mild disease.

Liver failure

Occasionally those with liver failure wish to travel and all the precautions discussed above under immunocompromise are important. Medications and malaria prophylaxis will require specialist advice. Overindulgence in alcohol while overseas is very common and dangers must be made very clear. It is not uncommon to see travellers returning from holidays abroad experiencing signs of liver failure for the first time.

Epilepsy

Legal restrictions on driving vehicles and piloting aircraft are for safety reasons and the traveller should not be tempted to take chances in countries where legislation relating to epilepsy is more lax or not enforced. Activities such as swimming and sub-aqua sports can also be dangerous. Tiredness, jetlag, alcohol, and illness may all make uncontrolled epilepsy worse. Usual medication may not be easily obtained in some countries. Starting new, or discontinuing regular, medication can cause problems. This also applies to illicit drugs which may be more easily obtained overseas.

Malaria prophylaxis needs to be carefully considered. Both chloroquine and mefloquine have been occasionally associated with convulsions. Doxycyline is an alternative in areas with resistance.

HIV infection and AIDS

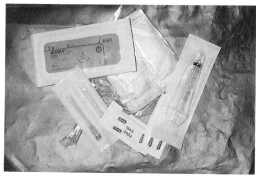

An HIV prevention pack.

Patients with HIV infection should take advice from their specialist before planning trips abroad especially to countries where the likelihood of contracting infections is high. For example, tuberculosis, salmonellosis, and cryptosporidial infections can all cause special problems for these patients.

In general, vaccinations, live or killed, can be given to HIV antibody positive persons at risk, although it may be prudent to use the killed poliomyelitis vaccine in symptomatic patients. BCG should not be given to symptomatic HIV carriers and should usually be withheld from those who are asymptomatic. Many countries have restrictions regarding the entry of HIV antibody positive persons and ask for blood tests before a visa is granted to long stay visitors or expatriates. The need for regular supervision must also be taken into account by this group of travellers; facilities may not be of the standards available at home and unusual or expensive medications be unavailable.

Diabetes mellitus

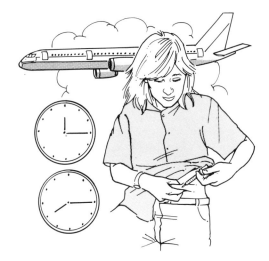

For short trips such as package holiday tours diet can be selected from normal menus. Emergency carbohydrate (sweets and starch) must be always available. Ample supplies of personal drugs, insulin, and testing equipment should be taken as new supplies obtained abroad may be initially difficult to identify because of different names, tablet sizes, and strengths.

Patients taking oral hypoglycaemic agents need not change their schedules even when crossing time zones.

Patients on insulin should have individual schedules worked out by their doctor. The following are general guidelines.

When crossing many time zones it is convenient for the diabetic to remain on home time for injections and carbohydrate intake until arrival. After that each insulin injection can be altered by two to three hours until they are fully adjusted to the new local time. If the time between injections is longer than usual a small supplementary injection of soluble insulin may be needed if urine tests become very sugary. If the time between injections is shorter than usual a small temporary decrease in dose may be advisable, perhaps 4 or 8 units. Often it will take a few days to re-establish normal control and the need for urine or capillary blood sugar estimations every four to six hours over this period must be emphasised.

Disposable syringes are unbreakable and safe to reuse without cleaning with spirit even in the tropics. A few should be kept in hand luggage. Cooling of insulin is not essential for short trips (see table). Insulin should never be carried in luggage that is put in the hold of an aircraft, as it must not be frozen.

Insulin must be continued during diarrhoeal or other illnesses, and the patient should also take easily absorbable carbohydrate. If vomiting occurs injections should continue and hospital care be sought. Ketoacidosis is rare in some races living in the tropics so the experience of local doctors may be limited. The accustomed facilities for managing eye, renal, and neuropathic complications may also be unavailable. Companions should be aware of the condition. Advice on medical insurance is available from the British Diabetic Association (see chapter on sources of advice).

Storage temperatures and shelf life of insulin

	Months of acceptability	
Temperature of store (°C)	Soluble insulin	Intermediate insulin
20	62	90
30	13	11
40	3	1·5
45	1·5	0·6

Other conditions

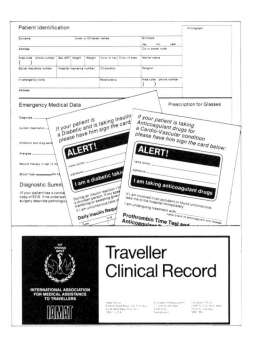

Renal calculi—Despite attempts to maintain a high urine flow, people with renal calculi tend to suffer worse symptoms in hot climates. If symptoms are severe or frequent and there is no treatable cause such as hyperparathyroidism or gout they will be exacerbated by long periods in the tropics.

Musculoskeletal disorders—Many people find that aches and pains of muscular or ligamentous origin improve in hot climates. Changes in lifestyle may be partly responsible. Ankylosing spondylitis tends to improve but the effect on rheumatoid arthritis is less predictable.

Lack of physical fitness—Activities such as skiing, swimming in the sea, or even sight-seeing can be very strenuous, and tiredness leads to accidents. Appropriate training before departure can be advised.

Obesity—Gross obesity can make life in the tropics difficult because of a greater tendency to heat exhaustion, excessive sweating, dermatitis, and skin infections.

Skin disorders—Psoriasis usually improves (it can be made worse by chloroquine) but severe eczema and acne are often worse in the tropics. Those already prone to skin infections will need to take special care. Excessive salt loss through the skin in cystic fibrosis can make heat adaptation more difficult.

Patient retained records in case of emergency

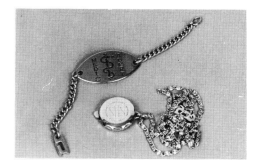

A traveller's clinical record containing a medical history including details of previous surgical operations and current drug treatment can be of great help to new medical attendants.

If a traveller has a serious allergy or is taking anticoagulants, steroids, insulin, or other drugs where regular doses are required and uncontrolled dosage or withdrawal is potentially dangerous, the problem can be displayed by carrying a card or wearing an engraved bracelet or necklace.

CHILDREN, WOMEN TRAVELLERS, THE ELDERLY, AND THOSE WITH A PHYSICAL DISABILITY

Travelling with children

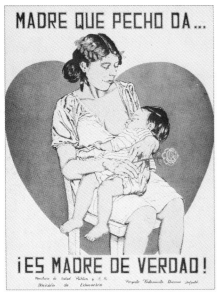

The generalisation that children travel well refers principally to their ability to enjoy new experiences. It must not be taken to mean that immunisations, preparation for travel, and other measures to prevent illness are less important than for adults. Children should be as fit as possible before departure, and this includes paying special attention to existing ailments and teeth. During air flights a contented child can prevent exhaustion of the parents, and if forewarned, most airlines can make special seating arrangements and provide cots for babies. They may also supply disposable nappies and special feeds, but it is wise to confirm this. At times a mild sedative such as chloral hydrate or an antihistamine during long flights is useful.

In many tropical countries child morbidity and mortality is much higher than in Britain. In general this does not apply to expatriates' children when they have adequate food, take care with hygiene, have received immunisations, and receive medical help early in illness. Medical facilities and the availability of drugs may, however, be wrongly taken for granted.

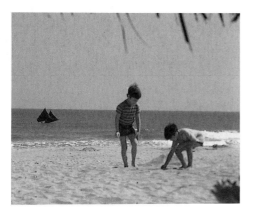

MADRE QUE PECHO DA...

¡ES MADRE DE VERDAD!

Breast is best.

Diet

It is wise to breast feed infants and it may be convenient to continue this for longer than is usual in Britain—even well into the second year of life. Feeding babies with fresh or reconstituted dried cows' milk provides them with opportunities for ingesting pathogenic organisms through the milk or from utensils; also the higher concentration of salt in unmodified cows' milk contributes to hyperosmolar dehydration, which can complicate gastroenteritis.

Local advice may be obtained about weaning foods. Millets, cereals, and pulses can all be ground and used. Although convenient, tins of baby foods may be expensive and not necessarily more nutritious. Care must, however, be taken to avoid contamination during preparation, and in general feeds should be used immediately and not stored. Bacterial contamination develops more rapidly when the atmosphere is humid. Green vegetables and fruits are important to provide vitamins A and C.

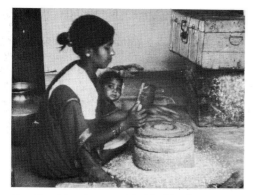

Unrefined foods protect babies' teeth.

Teeth

Breast feeding encourages normal development and positioning of teeth. When children are unlikely to ingest enough fluoride—that is, 1 part per million in water—to protect their teeth from caries fluoride tablets should be considered. Additional fluoride is more likely to be needed if surface water is drunk than if the water comes from artesian or deep wells. The amounts of fluoride contained in fluoride tablets or drops as prescribed in Britain are unlikely to do harm even when natural fluoride is present in the water, except in very young children in whom too much fluoride can cause mottling of the teeth. In an increasing number of countries it is now possible to find out the fluoride concentrations of public water supplies.

Before travelling
  General health
  Immunisations

During stay
  Balanced diet
  Care with preparation of food
  Good hygiene
  Avoid bites
  Malaria prophylaxis
  Seek medical help early

Climate

The long term effects of climate on children are difficult to assess because many other influences such as social, economic, dietary, and infective factors are involved. Although practices like placing a baby in a pram in the tropical sun must be avoided, a hot climate itself seems to do little harm to healthy children from temperate areas. Nevertheless, maintaining salt balance and avoiding sunburn are important. Prickly heat is more a problem in children than in adults.

Immunisation and malarial prophylaxis

When children are overseas it is wise to review immunisation procedures in the light of the practices of the host country. Diphtheria, pertussis, tetanus, and polio vaccinations can be begun in the first month of life when these diseases are widespread. Measles vaccine can be given from 6 months and again at 15 months of age (as MMR) in regions where measles, because of its high prevalence, tends to infect children as soon as their maternally acquired immunity has waned. BCG can be given from birth and prevent miliary or meningitic forms of tuberculosis in infants. Hepatitis B vaccine can also be given from birth and vaccines against meningitis (meningococcal, *Haemophilus influenzae*) and Japanese B encephalitis should be given if indicated. Typhoid vaccine is normally withheld until 1 year of age. Hepatitis A vaccine is now licensed for use in children and gives prolonged protection. For reasons not altogether clear, severe malaria is unusual in babies during the first few months of life, but expatriates should give malarial prophylaxis to their children from birth.

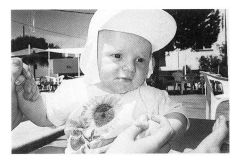

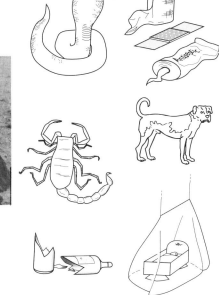

Accidents and bites

As children begin to crawl and walk they become more vulnerable to faecal–oral infections and hazards such as bites, accidents, and burns. Open wounds should be kept clean and covered with dressings until healed. Deaths from scorpion bites are unusual but mostly occur in children aged under 2 years. Allowing toddlers to play outside unattended can be particularly hazardous.

Taking adequate malarial prophylaxis should not encourage the traveller to ignore the risks from other mosquito borne diseases such as dengue, which can be more severe in children. Protection from mosquito bites is also important in those children who are strongly allergic to them. Appropriate clothes and cot plus window netting are usually more valuable in the long term than insect repellents.

Women travellers

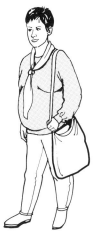

When travelling, women may have to consider menstruation, pregnancy, contraception, and also the possibility of sexual attack. Sanitary aids may not be available. Lack of toilets or privacy may lead to embarrassment, for example, on long bus journeys. Simple adaptations like wearing long dresses can help if it is necessary to use the road side. Advice from experienced local female friends can be helpful.

The stress of travelling can lead to menstrual irregularities and menstrual problems such as pain or menorrhagia may be more inconvenient. Advice should be sought well before departure if necessary. Fluid retention during menstruation is more likely in hot climates.

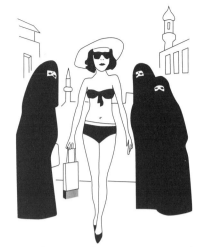

Women travellers—not humorous: woman in mini skirt or otherwise scantily dressed walking down a street in a Moslem country, attracting attention, where other women are fully veiled.

Remember:

- Live vaccines—avoid if possible
- Consider tetanus toxoid
- Immunoglobulin for hepatitis A
- Malaria prophylaxis

Oral contraceptives:

- Available locally?
- Can be taken continually during travel
- May contribute to fluid retention

Condoms:

- May be difficult to obtain
- Quality?
- Storage?
- Give some protection against sexually transmitted diseases

Fear of attack discourages many women, quite reasonably, from travelling alone. Points to remember are to plan routes, destinations, and accommodation with care, respect local customs and dress accordingly. In hot countries most locals cover up and avoid the sun. Do not encourage harassment by displaying expensive jewellery. Cheerful children can be cover for pickpockets.

Pregnancy

The general health of the mother, her previous obstetric history, and the facilities for managing complications and giving blood transfusions should all be taken into account when planning a pregnancy overseas. If antenatal care is carried out overseas but the mother plans to return to Britain for the delivery it must be remembered that most airlines do not allow passengers to travel after 35 weeks of pregnancy.

Live vaccinations are best not given during pregnancy though if someone unprotected against yellow fever is going to live in a high risk area, the theoretical risk of vaccination is outweighed by the serious nature of the illness. If a certificate of vaccination is required a doctor's letter endorsed with a health board or authority stamp to say the inoculation is contraindicated is usually accepted in its place, except when travelling from an infected to a non-infected zone. Inactivated poliomyelitis vaccine may be used instead of the usual oral live vaccine. Some manufacturers warn against the use of their inactivated vaccines although there is no clinical evidence of them causing harm.

A mother immunised against tetanus passes on protection to her baby over the neonatal period and a booster can be given during pregnancy if necessary. Hepatitis A in pregnancy may be more severe and also result in a prolonged prothrombin time and premature labour. Immunisation with immunoglobulin (the active vaccine is not licensed for use in pregnancy) should be encouraged.

Malarial prophylaxis should be maintained throughout pregnancy, as risks from most of the drugs normally used are less than the danger of malaria to the mother and fetus (see chapter on malaria).

Contraception

Those using oral contraceptives should be aware that absorption may be affected during gastrointestinal illnesses, that some brands may not be available locally, and that they may be continued over the usual break in the cycle if menstruation is going to occur at an inconvenient time such as during a long journey. They may contribute to the fluid retention that some people experience in hot climates, and they should not be taken by women suffering from hepatitis.

Condoms also give some protection against sexually transmitted diseases including HIV. The quality of those bought overseas may not be as good as expected, and storage can be a problem in very hot climates.

The elderly

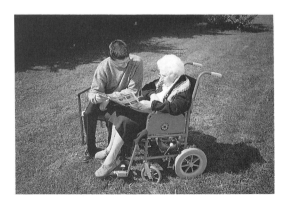

Age is no longer a bar to travelling abroad. Visiting relatives in New Zealand and Australia is common, and organised holidays to explore, for example, countries in Asia and South America are increasingly available. Cruises are very popular with the elderly. Some companies, such as SAGA, arrange holidays with the special needs of the elderly in mind, which may include special facilities for wheelchairs and bathing. Sometimes nursing and medical attention is on hand.

Advice given in other sections of this book on food and water hygiene, existing health problems, acclimatisation etc. must all be taken into account. Immunisations are just as important for the elderly as for younger people—age alone does not confer immunity.

Venous thrombosis during prolonged air flights is a particular risk and the need for moving around and exercises should be emphasised. Some would even suggest prophylaxis with subcutaneous heparin in those particularly predisposed. If there is a problem with bladder control it may be possible to arrange a seat near to a toilet, but on large aircraft toilets can become very busy and unpleasant to use towards the end of a long journey. Remember to arrange insurance which includes emergency repatriation.

Those with a physical disability

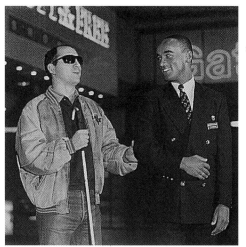
Courtesy of British Airways

Travel with a physical disability is now also commonplace, and adapting to unforeseen circumstances can be seen as a challenge. However, some advance knowledge of facilities available can be very important, especially for those with mobility problems. Airlines are often very helpful if given advance notice but over-booking and delayed flights may make assistance difficult. Facilities may be poor or absent in busy or smaller airports particularly in less developed countries.

Accommodation (ask about staircases), bathroom facilities, and special food requirements should be enquired about well in advance, although sometimes promises are not fulfilled. Modern buildings, although less "romantic" may have better facilities.

All the advice given elsewhere about preparations before travel applies to the disabled and comprehensive health insurance is important.

Extra advice can be obtained from the Royal Society for Disability and Rehabilitation (see chapter on sources of further information).

SOURCES OF FURTHER INFORMATION AND EDUCATION

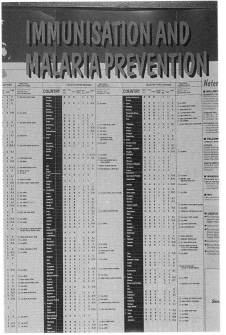

Wall charts can be very useful but are not an alternative to a sound consultation.

All overseas travellers need advice even if it is only of a strictly functional nature such as checking visa requirements or train departure times. Most will seek more information than this to try to predict difficulties and enhance their enjoyment. The information required will vary greatly from person to person, and the sources of information are equally diverse. These range from the vagaries of personal reminiscence, through the understandable bias of the travel industry to the remote detachment of the specialist centres. Such advice is profusely available in both verbal and written form.

The following lists are selective but include sources that are readily available and frequently updated. Advice on illnesses occurring after return can, in Britain, be obtained from local consultants in infectious diseases or tropical medicine.

Information from the Department of Health and the World Health Organisation

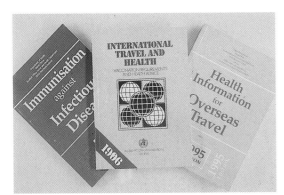

Official publications from WHO (centre) and the DoH (the "green book" on the left and the "yellow book" on the right).

Department of Health—The "T5" leaflet *Health Advice for Travellers*, (available free from post offices) is produced yearly and contains advice on reducing health risks and a list, by country, of compulsory and recommended immunisations. It advises about travel insurance and entitlement to medical treatment at reduced cost, and contains an application for certificate E111 (which entitles nationals of the European Union to care in other member states).

World Health Organisation, Geneva—International Travel and Health. Vaccination Requirements and Health Advice, yearly (available from HM Stationery Office). This lists by country compulsory immunisations and the risk of malaria and gives the distribution by geographical area of other health risks and appropriate preventive advice. It is aimed particularly at national health administrations and specialised advice centres and is not recommended for the individual traveller without medical knowledge.

Department of Health, Welsh Office, and Scottish Home and Health Department—Immunisation against Infectious Disease (the "green book") is produced in alternate years (HMSO) and is an invaluable source of reference and "official advice". *Health Information for Overseas Travel* (a "yellow book") first published in 1995, gives sound vaccination and malaria advice for different countries, some general principles of disease prevention, and includes a list of yellow fever vaccination centres in Britain. Its value will depend upon how often it can be updated.

Publications, specialist centres, concerned groups and professional societies

The International Society of Travel Medicine

The International Society of Travel Medicine has been established for about 8 years. It publishes the *Journal of Travel Medicine*, a newsletter and supports research. It organises a bi-annual international conference.

Secretariat: PO Box 871089, Stone Mountain, GA 30087-0028, USA.

Centres specialising in up to date medical advice for health care professionals only:

Scottish Centre for Infection and
  Environmental Health
Ruchill Hospital,
Glasgow G20 9NB   Tel: 0141 946 7120

PHLS Communicable Disease Surveillance
  Unit
61 Colindale Avenue
London NW9 5EQ   Tel: 0181 200 6868

Department of Communicable and Tropical
  Diseases,
Birmingham Heartland Hospital,
Bordesley Green Road,
Birmingham B9 5ST   Tel: 0121 766 6611

Department of Infectious Diseases and
  Tropical Medicine,
Monsall Hospital,
Manchester M10 8WR   Tel: 0161 205 2393

Hospital for Tropical Diseases,
180–2 Tottenham Court Road,
London W1P 9LE   Tel: 0171 637 9899

Liverpool School of Tropical Medicine,
Pembroke Place,
Liverpool L3 5QA   Tel: 0151 708 9393

Centres providing travel health advice directly to the travelling public at a charge include:

The Medical Advisory Service for Travellers (MASTA), based at the London School of Hygiene and Tropical Diseases, Keppel Street, London WC1E 7HT (0171 631 4408). Health briefs are provided in response to the travellers' details given by recorded message.

Pre-recorded health advice by country is available from the Hospital for Tropical Diseases in London (0898 345081) or from the Liverpool School of Tropical Medicine (0891 172111).

Regular publications

The Journal of Travel Medicine and a society "NewsShare" are published quarterly by the International Society of Travel Medicine (see box below).

Travelling Healthy is a simple but very informative bi-monthly publication alerting travellers and professionals to health and medical issues.
(Editor: 108–48, 70th Road, Forest Hills, New York, NY 11375)

Travel Medicine International is a journal aimed at doctors and nurses involved in travel medicine issues.
(Publishers: Mark Allen, Croxted Mews, 288 Croxted Rd, London SE24 9BY)

Wilderness and Environmental Medicine is the journal of the Wilderness Medical Society.
(Publishers: Chapman & Hall, 115 Fifth Avenue, New York, NY 10003)

Green Globe is a worldwide environmental management and public awareness programme aimed at the travel and tourism industry.
(Secretariat: 20 Grosvenor Place, London SW1X 7TT)

Doctor and *Practice Nurse* journals, *MIMS* and *Pulse* publish charts of recommended and compulsory immunisations plus advice on malaria risk. These are readily available in surgeries and are updated regularly. Because of conciseness they tend to be inflexible in relation to a traveller's lifestyle but can be a useful first source of reference so long as outdated copies are discarded.

Useful reference books for the health care professional
Diseases of Infection. NR Grist *et al.*, Oxford University Press, 1994, 019262307
Useful chapters on Imported Infections (14), Infection in the Tropics (15), and Prevention of Infection: Immunisation and Advice to Travellers (16).

Control of Communicable Disease Manual. AS Benenson *et al.*, APHA, 1995, 087553077X
An invaluable source of reference on common and unusual infections, published by the American Public Health Association.

MIMS (Monthly Index of Medical Specialties). Haymarket Medical, Tel: (44) 171 938 0705
Regularly updated lists of medical products available in UK. Special section on travel vaccines and malaria prophyaxis.

Sports Medicine. GR McLatchie, Churchill/Livingstone, 1993, 0443048746
Valuable source of information on prevention and management of injuries which may be related to travel, including exposure.

Travel Associated Disease. G C Cook (ed.), Royal College of Physicians, 1995, 1860160123
Reports of a symposium held in June 1994 at the London College of Physicians.

Healthy Skin—The Facts. R Mackie, Oxford University Press, 1992, 0192622447
The short section on sun and the skin is especially useful.

British National Formulary. BMA/RPS
(6 monthly), 0853692563
One of the essential desktop books for those prescribing drugs and vaccines in the UK.

Manson's Tropical Diseases. GC Cook *et al.* (eds), Saunders, 1996, 0702017647
The "Bible" of tropical diseases—an invaluable reference source, providing answers to all those difficult questions.

Lecture Notes on Tropical Diseases. D Bell, Blackwell, 1991, 0632024550
An excellent introduction to tropical diseases, both clinical aspects and prevention.

Travel and Health in The Elderly. IB McIntosh, Quay, 1992, 1856420698
A comprehensive guide that also has helpful advice for younger disabled travellers.

On line databases

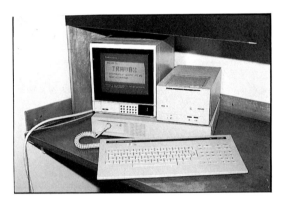

On line computerised databases have the advantage of immediate updating. TRAVAX, a system provided within the National Health Service, is available to general practitioners and others from the Scottish Centre for Infection and Environmental Health, Ruchill Hospital, Glasgow G20 9NB (Tel: 0141 946 7120). It gives information on vaccinations, malaria prevention and other health risks and is used in preparing the charts in *Practice Nurse, Doctor* and *Pulse*. MASTA (see above) provides a database to British Airways travel clinics and other commercial outlets.

A useful source of information on the WorldWideWeb is available via: http://www.cdc.gov and is compiled by the Center for Disease Control, Atlanta, USA.

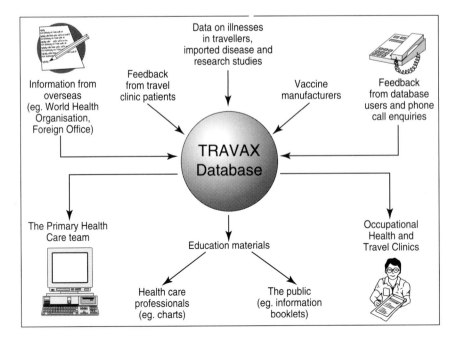

How travel information systems work.

Specialist associations

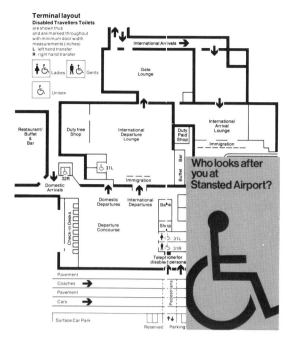

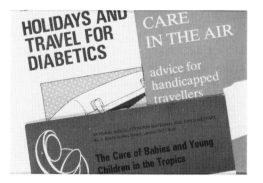

Many specialist associations produce booklets or leaflets, or provide services in connection with the problems of travel or life abroad. Addresses where these may be obtained are given.

Air Transport Users Committee, 1229 Kingsway, London WC2B 6NN (0171 242 3882) *Care in the Air*, advice for handicapped travellers.

British Airways Medical Service, Queens Building (N121), Heathrow Airport, Hounslow, Middlesex (0181 526 7070). *Your Patient and Air Travel*, useful booklet for medical practitioners with advice on fitness to travel and specific contraindications.

British Diabetic Association, 10 Queen Anne Street, London W1M 0BD (0171 323 1531). Leaflets and information, including *Travel Guide* to the more popular countries visited abroad, with advice pertinent to the needs of diabetics.

Intermedic, 777 Third Avenue, New York NY 10017, USA. A list of recommended English speaking doctors in many countries is available to members.

International Association for Medical Assistance to Travellers, Gotthardstrasse 17, 6300 Zug, Switzerland. Membership (free but voluntary contributions welcome) brings a directory of English speaking doctors and leaflets on climate, acclimatisation, immunisation, etc.

National Association for Maternal and Child Welfare, 1 South Audley Street, London W1Y 6JS (0171 383 4115). *The Care of Babies and Young Children in the Tropics*, by D Morley. *Travelling with Children*.

The Royal Association for Disability and Rehabilitation (RADAR), 25 Mortimer Street, London W1N 8AB (0171 250 3222). A wide range of leaflets and services are available to help the handicapped arrange, insure, and enjoy their travels.

Women's Corona Society, 274 Vauxhall Bridge Road, London SW1V 1BB (0171 828 1652). Provides advice and contacts for those travelling abroad in any capacity. Booklets and day courses on living overseas are available.

Foundation for Teaching Aids at Low Cost (TALC). Institute of Child Health, 30 Guilford Street, London WC1N 1EH. A list is available of books and pamphlets for purchase, primarily for medical and paramedical workers concerned with health problems in the Third World.

Travel agent sources

Did they mention malaria?

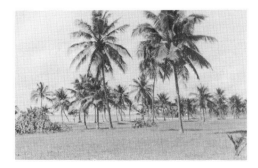

Travel agents, though having a responsibility to make clients aware of all risks, do not normally highlight them as they do other aspects of their holidays. Many directories are available to the travel trade that give regular up to date information on visa requirements, recommended immunisations, currency and customs allowances, and climate country by country. Examples are the *Travel Information Manual*, published monthly by the International Air Transport Association (subscriptions from TIM, PO Box 7627, 1118 zj, Schiphol Airport, The Netherlands), the *ABC Guide to International Travel*, published quarterly (subscriptions from ABC Travel Guides Ltd, World Timetable Centre, Dunstable, Bedfordshire LU5 4HB), and *World Travel Guide*, published yearly by Columbus Press, which is probably the most comprehensive of the three but is expensive.

Travel agents will readily pass on this information but they cannot usually interpret different risks for individual travellers flexibly, so again the advice tends to become dogmatic. Increasingly pressure is being put upon travel agents to take more responsibility for the health of their clients and some travellers' claims for negligence have been successful.

General sources of advice and information aimed at travellers

Some advice from the host countries

A group of Asian Christians, meeting at a consultation arranged by the Christian Conference of Asia in 1983 offered these suggestions to guide tourists.

- Travel in a spirit of humility and with genuine desire to learn more about the people of your host country. Be sensitively aware of the feelings of other people, thus preventing what might be offensive behaviour on your part. This applies very much to photography.
- Cultivate the habit of listening and observing, rather than merely hearing and seeing.
- Realise that often the people in the country you visit have time concepts and thought patterns different from your own. This does not make them inferior, only different.
- Instead of looking for that "beach paradise" discover the enrichment of seeing a different way of life through other eyes.
- Acquaint yourself with local customs. What is courteous in one country may be quite the reverse in another—people will be happy to help you.
- Instead of the Western practice of "knowing all the answers", cultivate the habit of asking questions.
- Remember that you are only one of thousands of tourists visiting this country and do not expect special privileges.
- If you really want your experience to be a "home away from home", it is foolish to waste money on travelling.
- When you are shopping remember that "bargains" you obtained were only possible because of the low wages paid to the maker.
- Do not make promises to people in your host country unless you can carry them through.
- Spend time reflecting on your daily experiences, in an attempt to deepen your understanding. It has been said that "what enriches you may rob and violate others".

Any comments or reactions to this code of ethics can be sent to the Ecumenical Coalition on Third World Tourism, PO Box 10–1014, Bangkok 10311, Thailand.

Useful reference books for the more adventurous travelling public

Traveller's Health—How to Stay Healthy Abroad. R Dawood, Oxford University Press, 1992, 0192618318
Useful for the traveller who wants to be well informed or as a reference for health care professionals.

The "Rough Guide" Series. Various authors and dates, Harrap Columbus
Travel guides aimed at the adventurous traveller. They contain some health information of varying quality. Useful example of information available to the general public.

Health, Hazard and the Higher Risk Traveller. IB McIntosh, Quay, 1993, 1856420817
A valuable look at the problems facing travellers with pre-existing health problems or undertaking "risky" activities such as water sports, high altitude treks and expeditions.

Bugs, Bites and Bowels. JW Howarth, Globe Pequot, 1995, 0860110452
An informed, chatty book based on personal experience. A useful example of information available to the general public.

Good Health Good Travel (previously *Health beyond Heathrow*). Ted Lankester, Interhealth, 1993, 0952164000
Especially useful health guide for volunteers and expatriates working overseas.

Travel in Health. G Fry and V Kenny, International Safari, 1994, 0952293900
Aimed at the traveller, an easily read and accurate common-sense guide.

Globe-trotter's Bible. Katie Wood, Harper Collins, 1996, 0006386881
A personalised guide to budget travel around the world. A useful reference for details about individual countries. Not a lot on health.

Handbook for Women Travellers. M and G Moss, Piatkus, 1995, 0749914394
A valuable look at the particular problems that may face women travellers from health issues to harassment.

Education in travel medicine

Do not over-simplify the pre-travel consultation

Vaccine charts are not a substitute for sound risk assessment and advice on lifestyle

Some knowledge of natural history of diseases unusual in Britain is required

Seek advice if in doubt about illness in those returning from abroad

Opportunities for education in travel medicine are increasing. In Britain initiatives have focussed upon general practice and in particular practice nurses, who take on much of the practical work of advising travellers.

There is a course leading to a Diploma in Travel Medicine awarded by the University of Glasgow in conjunction with the Scottish Centre for Infection and Environmental Health. It is open to qualified doctors and nurses with relevant experience and is a one-year distance learning course combined with residential periods. Students study in detail topics similar to those covered in this book and complete a mini-project. Successful candidates can continue onto a substantial research project leading to an MSc. A short introductory certificated course is also offered which uses core material from the Diploma.

Enquiries to: Susan Harvey (course secretary), Ruchill Hospital, Bilsland Drive, Glasgow G20 9NB. Tel: 0141 946 7120.)

Topics included in the Diploma in Travel Medicine at Glasgow University

Historical aspects of travel medicine
Infections spread by food, water, soil, insects, animals, and personal contact
Immunisation theory and available vaccines
Malaria prevention and treatment
Problem travellers and fitness to travel
Injuries associated with travel (physical, solar, physiological, baro-trauma)
Sexually transmitted diseases
Sources of travel information: running a travel clinic
Illness in the returned traveller
Women travellers: child travellers
Psychiatric aspects of travel and living abroad
Altitude: winter sports injuries
Aeromedical evacuation: expedition medicine
Protracted visits (e.g. expatriates and missionary work)
Policies, protocols, and legal aspects

There is also a home learning course in travel medicine for practice nurses organised by the "Magister" Nurse Open Learning programme. This involves study units and assignments. Enquiries to: Freepost BS 9133, Frome, Somerset BA11 1YA.

These courses, in addition to improving day to day travel medicine practice, should help those qualified to develop teaching skills in the specialty and encourage an interest in surveillance and research.

The enclosed chart is updated every 3 months and copies are made available regularly in *Practice Nurse* and *Doctor* magazines. It is sponsored by SmithKline Beecham, whose representative can also provide updated copies, but the information is prepared independently by the Scottish Centre for Infection and Environmental Health.

INDEX

Index